I0571694

Code Blue Murder

Ashton Community Hospital, Volume 1

Nanci Race

Published by MFM Books, 2025.

Table of Contents

Dedication

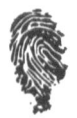

THIS BOOK IS DEDICATED to the hardworking crew of nurses at the Andrews House. You know who you are. You are the ones who inspired me to write this series.

Chapter One

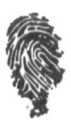

T he double doors of the Emergency room slid closed with a whoosh. The receptionist rose from her desk when no one approached. She walked around the counter and opened the door separating her from the waiting room. Peering around the corner, she noticed no one was there. *How odd. Maybe I'm imagining things. Did I really hear the doors?* Kylie thought she heard a whoosh but the sounds distorted when the separating door closed. Kylie Nichols walked back to her desk just as an ambulance backed into the ambulance bay.

She picked up the phone on her desk and pushed the first button. The response was immediate.

"Janessa Williams."

"Ash County ambulance is here," Kylie announced.

"Thanks, they're right on time. We're all set."

THE PARAMEDICS WHEELED the gurney into the emergency room of Ashton Community Hospital.

On the gurney lay a pale, blonde-haired woman. She was thin, almost to the point of emaciation. Janessa noted the blue tinge to her lips and nail beds as she was transferred to the bed in room one, the cardiac room in the emergency department. She lay unmoving, either not having the strength or not caring to look around at her surroundings.

"Lara, can you hear me? I'm Janessa Williams. I'll be your nurse for the evening. I'm going to put an IV, an intravenous line into your arm. That will make it easy for us to give you fluids and medications and draw blood for tests. Can you tell me what happened to you today?" Janessa badged into the computer and pulled up Lara Scutterby's history. "I see that you were here about three weeks ago for abdominal pain. That resolved itself a few hours after you came in so you were sent home. Is that why you came in today? Is the pain back?"

"No," Lara replied in a faint voice. Janessa strained to hear when the woman finally answered. Her voice was just above a whisper. "I just feel unwell. Same as always."

"Ok, Lara. I'll get that IV started. I see that your next of kin and healthcare proxy is your father. Do you want us to call him?"

"Don't!" The word reverberated throughout the room.

Terry Meyers, the other nurse on duty pushed the curtain aside and rushed into the room. "Everything okay in here? Do you need any help, Janessa?"

Janessa finished setting up the tray for the IV she needed to put into Lara's arm. "Thanks, Terry, we're fine. Lara was just emphasizing that she didn't want to worry her father with a call from us at this time."

"Old bastard won't be worried. He'd just as soon I die and get it over with. He'll be happy then. I won't be a drain on him when that happens. He's ignored me for years, so why would this time be any different?" She paused. "So no, don't call him. I'm 36 years old. As long as I'm in my right mind, he doesn't need to be here." She turned her head to see Janessa better. "Are you new here? I don't remember seeing you before."

"I usually work in the Critical Care Unit, but they had only one patient so two nurses don't need to be there at the moment and the emergency room was busy earlier in the evening. Let's get you settled and run tests to see what's going on. The Physician's assistant Darryl Mintz will be in to see you in a little while. I'll put these leads on you so we can monitor your heart and pulse rates, then I'll put in your IV so we can get fluids into you. Do you have any pain?"

Lara nodded. "Yes, there's a dull ache in the right side of my chest."

"We can probably give you something to ease the pain after Darryl has seen you. On a scale of one to ten how bad is it?"

"Seven," Lara stated without hesitating.

"Okay, I'll let Daryl know." Janessa finished inserting the intravenous line and checked the monitor reading of Lara's blood pressure and oxygen level. After she took an electrocardiogram to see how Lara's heart was functioning, she printed out a cardiac strip to show the physician's assistant when he came to see Lara. "I'll be right back, Lara. Try to rest. We'll take good care of you. Nothing to worry about."

Janessa left the room making sure she pulled the privacy curtain closed. She grabbed the nearest chair in the nurse's station and faced Terry. "I see that Lara is a frequent flyer." This was the unprofessional term many nurses and doctors used for patients who frequented the Emergency Department for one reason or another. "Drug seeker?"

Terry shrugged. "Not that I know, but with her, it's hard to tell. She's always in for something or other but she doesn't come right out and ask for drugs. My opinion? She's a Daddy attention seeker. She always has an ailment, but her father could care less. He rarely shows up to see her when she comes in with her various aches and pains."

"What do you mean? Is her father someone special?"

"Janessa, how long have you worked here? I thought you knew; her father is Leo Scutterby, the President of the Board of Directors of this hospital."

Janessa digested this information without replying. *That might explain why she doesn't want him notified. I've heard he's a real hardnosed businessman who doesn't tolerate fools.* The ding and whoosh of machines droned in the background while the nurses concentrated on paperwork. Janessa checked on Lara who appeared to be sleeping. Walking back to the nurse's desk she found the physician's assistant, Darryl Mintz sitting at the computer looking through Lara's records from previous visits.

"Hey, Janessa. No patients in Critical Care this evening?"

"There was one gentleman with acute chest pain, but Lila Warren is working, and she can manage things. The emergency room was busy, so the shift director asked me to come and help. Many of the patients were discharged so it's quieter."

"Glad you're here. Dr. Travis is on duty, and I expect he'll pop in a little later to examine Lara Scutterby. In the meantime, let's run the standard tests. We'll get the usual blood panel and chest x-ray then we'll take it from there. I see that her oxygen saturation level is down. Did you put her on oxygen?"

"Yes, she's on three liters. She complained of right-sided chest pain, which she says is a seven out of ten on the pain scale. Do you want her to have anything for pain?"

"Let's wait until we get the chest x-ray and some of the blood results. That shouldn't take long. I don't want to give her anything until then." He looked at the EKG printout that Janessa handed him. "Her EKG is showing a few PVCs, but otherwise it looks normal. Let's talk to Lara."

Janessa and Daryl parted the curtain into the cubicle where Lara lay, unmoving. When they got close to the gurney, she rolled over to look at them. Janessa noted that Lara winced and put her hand to her chest when she moved.

"Lara, I'm the physician's assistant, Darryl Mintz. I want to listen to your chest for a minute. Is that okay?"

At Lara's nod, he placed his stethoscope on her chest and moved it around to various places. He helped her sit up so he could listen to her lungs from her back. "Done. You can lie back now. Can you show me where you have pain?" He watched as she placed a hand just above her right breast. He manipulated areas around her abdomen, stood and smiled at the patient. "We're going to run tests then we'll decide on a course of treatment. Your EKG showed a few premature ventricular contractions or PVCs, but I don't think there's much to worry about. Until we get more test results, just rest."

Janessa and Daryl left the cubicle. He wrote the orders for the tests in Lara's chart, then left the nurse's station. She checked his orders and made notes in the electronic chart of all the procedures she had done so far. Fifteen minutes later the cardiac alarm blared a loud warning. Sometimes movement triggered the alarm, so Janessa wasn't worried. However, as she approached the gurney Janessa could see that something was very wrong. Lara wasn't breathing.

Chapter Two

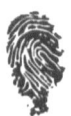

"Are you okay?" Janessa tapped Lara's shoulders and called to her. She checked for a pulse on the side of Lara's neck. *Nothing.* She adjusted the bed and began chest compressions. "Terry," she shouted, "get the crash cart and call a code. Lara's in cardiac arrest." As she continued pushing on Lara's chest, Janessa vaguely heard the overhead page. *"Code Blue, Emergency Room."*

It seemed like forever to Janessa, but it was actually minutes before the room was full of people. The code team, consisting of Dr. Travis, the emergency room doctor, Darryl Mintz, the physician's assistant, Terry, wheeling in the crash cart with all the drugs and equipment they would need, the IV team, that would put in more IV's and monitor them as meds were given and a host of other people. Someone inserted a tube into Lara's lungs so they could use an ambu bag to breathe for her. The nurse operating the defibrillator and heart monitor adjusted the dials while someone began recording all the medications and the entire process of every measure taken to save Lara's life.

As soon as the defibrillator charged the operator yelled, "Clear! All Clear!" She then pushed the button on the machine to administer a shock to Lara's heart. The woman's body jerked with each subsequent shock, but there was no return to a normal heart rhythm.

Forty-five minutes later, Dr. Travis said, "Time of death, 1940 hours."

Lara had been in the emergency room less than three hours. Now she was dead. Janessa began picking up tubing and syringes for disposal after she made sure the nurse recording everything catalogued them. She noted Terry's stiff movements and felt the same. It seemed surreal.

Thirty minutes ago, Lara was awake, aware, and talking. What had happened in that short amount of time?

"Terry?" The other nurse stopped what she was doing and looked across the room at Janessa. "Has anyone called Mr. Scutterby?" Janessa asked.

"Lara didn't want us to call him, remember, but someone sure needs to call him now," Terry answered. "God knows what the fallout from this will be. I hope someone has answers for him. I'll go tell Darryl that he or Dr. Travis needs to call Mr. Scutterby now. I'll be right back to help you finish cleaning up Lara. He might want to see her so we should remove all the tubes and the airway. No one should see their child like this."

After Terry left the room, Janessa began removing the tape holding the airway in place in Lara's mouth and took the intubation tube out. Then she removed the tape from Lara's arm and removed the port and IV. Janessa retrieved a wet, warm facecloth and gently wiped blood and mucous off Lara's face. She looked up when Terry entered the room.

"Darryl called Mr. Scutterby and gave him the bad news. Be prepared, he wants to see his daughter and he's really pissed that no one contacted him when she came into the ED. Darryl tried to explain that she requested he not be notified, but I could hear him screaming at Darryl on the phone. He wants to know what happened to her and who is responsible for her death."

Janessa paused in the process of cleaning the deceased woman. "He can't seriously think that one of us is responsible for this." She made a sweeping gesture encompassing the bed with Lara on it. "We did our best to take care of her and figure out the problem. I guess when you lose someone like this, especially your child, you need someone to blame even when you know deep down no one's at fault."

"There will be an autopsy, even if he doesn't insist on one."

"You think so?" Janessa was silent for a moment. "You're probably right. Her death does seem odd. There really is no medical reason that we know, yet. We don't have any test results, so we don't know anything really. I bet he'll insist on an autopsy. That way if it comes back that she didn't die of natural causes, he'll have someone to blame. Probably me since she was my patient."

A sudden commotion at the door caused the two nurses to look toward the curtained entryway. Janessa knew without a doubt that Leo Scutterby had arrived.

"Who is it? I want to know who's responsible for my daughter's death. Don't you people know what you're doing? She was 34 and had few medical issues. Who did this to her? My daughter is dead, and I want answers now!"

Janessa strode through the nurse's station to the outer part of the emergency room where Lara's father stood. Leo Scutterby was a big man. He looked to be about 6'4 " and probably weighed 260 pounds or more. Rather than grief-stricken, he looked angry. His fists clenched and unclenched at his side. "She was 36, sir. Lara was 36 years old. Mr. Scutterby, why don't we go into the office and talk?"

"Whatever. 34 or 36 it doesn't matter. She's dead and I don't want to talk," he shouted. "I want to know who killed my daughter. I'm President of the Board of Directors of this hospital. I'm entitled to know what happened to my child."

Janessa turned toward the room used as an office by the Nursing Director of the Emergency Room. She glanced over her shoulder and was satisfied to see that Leo Scutterby was following her. There were patients in the Emergency Room, sick patients who didn't need to hear the rantings of this man. She wanted to believe it was his grief making him so belligerent, but she doubted it. They reached the office, where she ushered Lara's father inside and closed the door behind them. While not soundproof, the closed door would cut down on the noise the patients could hear.

When the man sat in the chair on the opposite side of the desk from Janessa, she opened her mouth to tell him the circumstances of his daughter's death. Before she could utter a word, he half stood and jabbed a finger at her nearly touching her face.

"Who was taking care of her?" he demanded. His strident tone hadn't diminished since they'd entered the office. "My girl has always had minor issues, but she wasn't sick enough to die. Someone did something to her. Who was the doctor? I want to talk to him. Were you in the room with her? Were *you* her nurse?"

"Mr. Scutterby. Please sit down so that we can talk."

"My daughter is dead. I want answers. No woman her age comes into an emergency room and is dead just over an hour later. That other nurse said she hadn't been here long."

"That's right. She was here for approximately three hours. Now, if you'll sit down, I'll explain as best I can. We were trying to figure out what happened to your daughter. I understand how hard it is to lose a child no matter their age. I..."

"I don't want your platitudes; I want to know what happened to my only child. Do you have any children?"

Janessa shook her head and tried to continue. "I was her nurse. We were preparing to do tests. I drew a couple of vials of blood for blood tests. Your daughter stated she had pain in her upper right chest, so the physician's assistant ordered tests that might be more conclusive before we gave her anything for pain... He..."

"Physician's Assistant? They don't have medical degrees. Where was the on-call doctor? Why wasn't he taking care of her?"

"The doctor was with a critical patient at that time. Our Physician's Assistants are extremely well trained, as I'm sure you know. We were waiting for test results to come back before we decided on a course of treatment. I put an IV in Lara and gave her fluids through the IV then drew blood for the other tests. Shortly after we finished taking an EKG, Lara told us about the pain she was having, and the prudent course of action was to wait for the test results so that we could see what we were dealing with. At that point, we didn't know if there was a physical cause for her illness or if something else was going on."

"Something else going on? What's that supposed to mean?" Leo Scutterby stood and slammed the chair back until it crashed into the wall behind him. "What else do you think was going on? Psychosomatic illness? Drugs?" He was so agitated that flecks of spittle shot from his mouth onto the desk in front of him.

Janessa stood as well. "I said nothing about drugs or mental illness. We were trying to rule out all causes." The tone of her voice left no room for argument. "I think you've said enough, Mr. Scutterby. I'm sorry your daughter died, but we did our best. Now, if you'll excuse me, I have patients to take care of." The discussion was over.

He stepped back as Janessa brushed past him and opened the door. She glanced at him and noted his heavy breathing and mottled red face. She sent up a silent prayer that he wouldn't keel over from a stroke on her watch.

"We're not done. You'd better get all your ducks in a row because if I find out that my daughter's death was because of your negligence, I'll make sure the nursing board permanently pulls your license. The only job you'll get in any hospital will be cleaning the toilets. Do I make myself clear? Do you hear me? I said I'm coming for you and your job if I find out you had anything to do with my daughter's death."

Janessa kept walking. Trying to talk to the man in the midst of his grief was impossible. Lara Scutterby was dead at 36 years old, but Janessa had done her best to take care of her. Second guessing her actions wouldn't do any good. It was too late for that.

Chapter Three

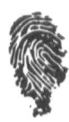

Days after Lara Scutterby's death, Janessa was working in Critical Care, her usual unit. Her co-worker and best friend Marguerite was also on duty. Their patients were settled so they sat at the nurse's station. The steady beep of the cardiac monitors hummed in the background, a signal that the patients' hearts were stable at that moment.

"Did Scutterby really threaten you?"

Janessa swiveled her chair so she could look fully at Margarite. "He said that if he found out I was responsible for his daughter's death he'd make sure I lost my license and that I'd be cleaning toilets in the hospital instead of nursing. I'm sure Bully Bill in HR would love that. I wish I could hear the conversation between him, Mr. Scutterby and Potts."

"Harsh," Margarite said with a grimace. "Tell me again what happened. I know you put in an IV and drew blood for testing. What happened between the time she came in and the time she died? She must have been sicker than everyone thought."

"Nothing really happened. That's what's puzzling me. The PA on duty was Darryl Mintz. He's good and very observant. He examined Lara. The only thing he said was that he didn't want to give her anything for pain until at least some test results came back. Her EKG showed a few PVCs but nothing notable about her cardiac rhythm."

"Pain?"

"Yes, she complained of pain in upper right chest. She had good respirations, and her saturation level was 95 percent after I put her on three liters of oxygen.

"Does her father want an autopsy?"

Janessa checked the monitor in front of her before answering. "He says he does. That's when he threatened to have my license pulled. I know I didn't do anything wrong. I'm meticulous about the care I give my patients. Lara Scutterby got the best care. However, if I was her father, I'd ask for one too. She was so young. None of it makes sense."

Margarite's green eyes widened as she gazed at Janessa. She couldn't conceal her anxiety. Janessa felt bad for frightening her friend, but Margarite was the only one she trusted.

"I know you. I know the type of nurse you are. I'm sure you gave her great care. You said earlier that she came to the Emergency Department quite often. Terry seemed to know her quite well. Didn't you say she told you that Lara was a frequent flyer? Maybe that's the problem. What are you going to do now?"

"She did tell me that, but she also stressed that she wasn't a drug seeker. Terry seems to think all Lara's complaints were to get her father's attention. Janessa stood and walked to the door leading into the patient's room. "She was there frequently, with no specific illness. No one comes into the ER that many times and has nothing wrong with them even if it's psychological. Every test she's had in the past has been negative, including all the psych tests. She wasn't a nut job. Anyway, I'm not going to sit back and wait to be prosecuted. I'm going sleuthing. That's what I'm going to do now."

"What do you mean?" Margarite asked.

"I need to investigate this. One way or another I'm going to find out who killed Lara Scutterby. I don't plan to sit back and take the blame for something I didn't do. One minute she was talking to me and complained of minor pain in her right chest. Not long after that she was dead. It doesn't make sense. Someone knows something and I plan to find out who and what. What worries me is that it could happen to another patient."

"So, you suspect murder?"

Janessa sighed. "Yes. I do. I just don't know how or why. I do know that Lara didn't *just* die."

"How do you plan to go about investigating? You're not a cop." Margarite said. Maybe you should leave it up to them. They are more equipped to handle things like this."

Janessa looked back over her shoulder at Margarite. She brushed back a curl that had worked its way loose from the topknot she'd fashioned this morning. "I could leave it up to the police, but my reputation is on the line. If Leo Scutterby has his way, my job and nursing license are at stake. I'm going to ask questions. Someone in the ER or someone connected to the dead woman did something that caused her death, and I know it wasn't me. We'll find out for sure when the autopsy results come back. There must be something in those results that will give us a clue about what happened. Her death wasn't from natural causes. I'm sure of that. Her bloodwork should be back soon. It will take longer for the autopsy, if there is one. The toxicology screen takes longer, but it's been a while. I'll be able to check Meditech and see her results before things get crazy with this case. If anyone questions why I've accessed her electronic health record I'll let them know that she was my patient and I have a right to look at her results. In the meantime, I'm going to start asking questions."

"Do you think anyone will be willing to talk to you?" At Janessa's affirmative nod, Margarite continued. "Okay. I want to help. I mean, I can't let you go through this alone. After all, I am your only friend here. I'm the one you can trust. Let me question PA Hottie."

"Who?" Janessa turned away from the patient's room she'd been about to enter.

"Darryl Mintz. He's hot and I..."

"He's also married. His wife just had their fifth kid."

"Damn! He's still hot though. I can see why she has five kids. I mean it. I want to help. This could be dangerous, and I don't think you should do it alone."

"All right. You can question Kylie Baker Nichols. She was at the desk. Maybe she heard or saw something while Terry and I were busy."

"Janessa?"

She turned to look at Margarite.

"What if the autopsy turns up nothing? What do we do then? I mean, even if it doesn't show anything other than a natural cause, what's next?"

"Let's not get ahead of ourselves. We'll keep looking for answers. I know it wasn't a death from natural causes. I also know people can have heart attacks or strokes at 36, but my gut tells me this was something else. Nothing in her preliminary test showed anything abnormal."

"Boy, all my gut ever says is, 'feed me.' Wish mine would say something else." She looked from Janessa's slim figure to her own slightly fuller body.

Janessa smiled. "You are a beautiful woman, Margarite. Men fall all over you because of your gorgeous mane of red hair, green eyes, and curves. I'm about as curvy as a stick. Nothing to hold on to as my ex-boyfriend Trey was fond of saying. That's why he's my ex. So, I don't think you have anything to worry about. And if you are worried about your weight, remember what my Mama always said..."

"What?" Margarite interrupted.

"Treadmills are not designed to be clothes hangers and yours definitely is. The only time I've seen it clear was when you bought it. You must have bought it for a reason. Start using it. You look perfect to me, but on the other hand you're my best friend and I love you no matter what you look like."

Margarite pulled a face that made her look like a gargoyle. "Even this?"

Janessa chuckled. "Even that, you ugly thing."

"You're right, I suppose," Margarite said as a red flush crept into her face. "By the way, do you think you'll be talking to Detective Halen?

He *is* the only detective in this town and I'm sure he'll be the first one here drooling all over you."

It was Janessa's turn to flush. "Stop. He does not drool all over me." *Not like I drool over him.* Janessa kept that thought to herself. There were things one didn't admit even to one's bestie.

"He does. I can hear him panting after you from 50 feet away. Why don't you put him out of his misery and go out with him.?"

Again, Janessa started to enter the patient's room. "Two reasons. One, we don't know if Lara's death is a murder or by a natural cause, so until we're certain her death is a homicide, he won't be coming here. And two," She paused. "he hasn't asked me."

"When he does ask you, give him a chance. After all, you'll be helping him solve a murder."

Chapter Four

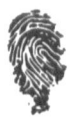

Janessa walked to the elevator and pressed the button for her floor. When it pinged and the doors opened, she walked off, rounded the corner to the left, and went through the double doors to the Critical Care Unit. Margarite was there, tending to the patients' notes on the computer, so Janessa had been able to go to the Emergency room to ask questions about Lara's death. Margarite had questioned people earlier, but the women hadn't had a chance to discuss her findings or any success she'd had getting people to talk to her.

"How did you make out?" Janessa asked her friend as she sat in the chair next to Margarite.

"I ran into several brick walls. No one saw or heard anything out of the ordinary. They either didn't see anything, they were oblivious, or they're just not saying. It's ridiculous. I mean, I'm not a cop. You'd think they wouldn't mind talking to me."

"Same here. Kylie says she thought she heard the sliding doors open and close. She looked but there was no one there. Five or ten minutes later she heard the same thing, but never saw anyone. So, what do you think?"

Margarite didn't answer right away. "Someone knows more than they're saying. They're either covering up for someone or they are the killer. As you said before, if it wasn't from natural causes, and I doubt it was, then someone helped her along to the great beyond. She certainly didn't kill herself. But" Margarite turned to scan the beeping monitor. "we don't even know if we have a murder yet. None of the tests are back so tell me again why we're investigating what, despite what you said before, might be a natural death?"

"Because I know in my gut it's a murder. We'll keep digging. There is a killer in this hospital, and we need to find him or her. If those tests and the autopsy come back that Lara's death was anything but natural, I'm the first one they'll look at. Lara's father has already accused me of doing something to his daughter, even though I had just met the woman. She was in the emergency department a lot, but that was the first time I'd worked there when she came into the place."

Margarite scooped her flame red hair into a top knot. "What did Terry have to say? She was on that night too. Did she see or hear anything? That woman is very strange."

"Nothing. But she said something odd, so I've been wracking my memory back to that night and her actions. She knew Lara from other visits, but she was almost hostile about her."

"What do you mean?" Margarite asked, turning to look fully at Janessa.

Janessa shrugged. "When I asked her if Lara was a drug seeker, she said not that she knew of, but then she said something about Lara being a Daddy attention seeker or something to that effect. Why would she say that? She was quite hostile about her. However, when I had her call the code for Lara's cardiac arrest, she was a complete professional."

"What did she mean? You're right, she sounds hostile. Wonder if she was jealous of Lara's wealth and privilege. That happens to the best of us sometimes you know."

"Hmmm, could be. But there was something else going on there. I couldn't get her to explain further, so I'm going to talk to her again later to see if she'll be any more forthcoming. It's obvious she didn't like Lara, but I can't figure out why. We've all had those patients who are not exactly our favorites, but this was different. Lara wasn't really a complainer and she seemed frightened. She was genuinely in pain from something."

"Terry was only in Lara's room when you were there, right?"

Janessa sighed. "Yes, as far as I know. That's what's so odd. Given Terry's hostility, I'd say she had a motive to get rid of Lara, but I didn't see her go into the room except when I was there. I stepped out briefly, but I don't think it was long enough for Terry to do anything. On the other hand, it only takes a few seconds to inject something into an IV port. I could be wrong about her hostility. Maybe it's a simple case of disliking someone you think is wasting hospital resources. First we need to find out if Lara died naturally or if someone murdered her. If you'll cover the unit, I want to go back down to the ER and dig around some more."

Margarite smiled. "You've got it Chief. I expect a full report when you come back. And Janessa?" Her friend turned to look at her. "Just be careful."

Janessa laughed. "I will, although I'm not sure what you think will happen to me in broad daylight with all the staff around."

"You never know. Someone could corner you in a supply room or something and hit you with a mop or a broom. You know what I mean. Lara was killed in the middle of a busy emergency department, so who knows. Just be careful."

"'Death by Mop,' what a way to go. I'll stay far away from the supply closets, I promise. The thought of a wet dirty mop over my head makes me gag. Especially if it's one that housekeeping uses in the bathrooms."

Margarite sniffed. "Okay, mock me. When you're tied up in a supply closet with a lump on your head and poop water dripping down your face, don't call me for help."

Janessa was laughing so hard at this point she doubled over. She tried to control herself so she wouldn't disturb the patients. "Girl, you should take up comedy. If I'm in a supply closet in the ER with a poopy mop on my head, I promise not to call you. Whoever the psycho is might come back and finish the job if they hear me calling you."

A short time later, Janessa looked at her watch and saw that it was her break time. "I'll be back shortly. I'm going to check Mr. Genow's vitals then I'm heading downstairs to tackle the beast."

"I'm not saying a word. You know my opinion on the matter. Don't know why you can't wait until we're off shift, then we can go together."

"Because, if we're off shift, where do you think Terry will be?"

"Oh. She'll be off, too. Just be careful. Besides..."

"You worry too much. I'll be fine. Now let me get these vitals so I can get down there."

Janessa finished with her patient in the Critical Care Unit, waved to Margarite, and headed for the elevator. She stepped off when she got to the floor that housed the Emergency Department. Unlike the sliding doors at the Emergency Room entrance, these glass doors automatically locked between the main part of the hospital and the ER and only accessible with a badge. She badged herself through and walked into the nurse's section of the Emergency Room. There was no sign of Terry, so she decided to wait and see if the other nurse returned.

Minutes later, Terry came around the corner and flopped into a chair beside Janessa. She fanned her face with a sheet of paper. "Wow, some procedures take the sweat right out of you. What are you doing here again, Janessa? Is it that slow in the unit? You were here earlier."

Janessa stared at Terry. The nurse was always friendly enough, but Janessa got a strange vibe from her, a vibe that made her uneasy. "It's not too bad up there. I wanted to follow up on our conversation about Lara Scutterby."

Terry frowned. The wrinkles in her brow remained despite a shallow smile. "She's dead and the world is a much better place. Give it up. People die every day."

"Aren't you concerned? She was so young, and the death was so sudden."

"Why should I be concerned? She wasn't my patient." Terry sneered at Janessa before looking away and busying herself with the papers on the desk. "If I were you, I would be worrying. Word around here is that Scutterby is out for blood, yours."

Janessa stood up to leave, knowing she wouldn't get any further with Terry. "He can be out for anything he wants. He's barking up the wrong tree if he comes after me. I'll just have to wait for the tox screen and autopsy report to come back," she said as she started to leave.

"They won't show anything."

Janessa stopped in her tracks and whirled around to look at Terry. "How do you know that?"

Terry waved her hand in Janessa's direction without looking up. "Go back upstairs. Nothing to see here, and I'm busy."

Janessa was thinking over the conversation with Terry when the elevator doors slid open, and she went around the corner through the doors to the Critical Care Unit. Margarite walked out of the patient's room and gave Janessa a pitying look. "Bully Bill in Human Resources wants you to call him. He's on the warpath and you can guess why."

Chapter Five

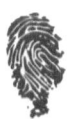

W illiam C. Magers III, better known by the staff as "Bully Bill," sat behind a large, shiny oak desk. The oversize desk matched his oversized body. Other than a picture of his wife and children, a huge desk calendar and a phone, the desk was clear. It was a decided testament to the amount of work he managed to do in a day. He smoothed a pudgy hand over the oak.

Finally. I can add to that know-it-all Janessa's file. I'll be rid of the little bitch with her superior attitude. I don't care who she is, she's gone too far this time. I hope Scutterby gets the cops to prove she's a murderer. At the very least she was careless with her patient. Ashton won't tolerate incompetence in a nurse.

He looked up when he heard the soft knock on his door. "Come in." He tried and failed to make his voice sound gruff and deep. Instead, what fell out of his mouth was a high-pitched squeak. When he was in high school, that had been his nickname, 'Squeaky.' He'd tried everything to change his voice. Gargling, deep breathing, endlessly clearing his throat. Nothing worked. Now, at 54 years old, he still sounded like someone's aged aunt with a bad cold.

Janessa Williams strode into his office and stood in front of his desk. He decided to make her squirm. He didn't ask her to sit in the chair opposite his desk until after he'd flipped through the papers in the folder several times. Five minutes passed before he looked up at Janessa. The smirk on her beautiful nut-brown face pissed him off even more.

"Sit!" He tried to force the word to come out deep and forceful. Instead, he had no control over the squeak that emanated from his vocal cords. He slammed the folder closed and sat back with his hands clasped. "Speak."

"I'm not a dog. Please don't talk to me and order me around as if I am one. I would say more, but I have no idea why you called me into your office. What seems to be the problem this time?" Without waiting for his reply, Janessa pulled out the chair across from his desk and sat down, defying him to tell her she couldn't.

William could feel the heat in his face, the beads of sweat dotting his forehead and upper lip. He pulled a pristine white handkerchief from his pocket and dabbed at his face. Satisfied that he had his emotions under control, he flipped open the folder once again.

"I understand you've been asking questions about the death of the patient, Lara Scutterby. You were her nurse. What don't you understand? She died. Her father blames you, and we're investigating the possibility that you were negligent."

It gratified him to see the look of horror on Janessa's face. This time he had her and with the backing of the president of the board. He was on a mission to prove that she was responsible for the patient's death. Come hell or high water, he would terminate her and make her pay for every slight and snide comment she'd ever made about him, as if he'd ever really wanted to date the little prude. Oh, he'd asked her, just like most of the single men in the facility when she'd first started working at Ashton Community. He still cringed when he thought about her response.

William had cornered Janessa in the elevator. Pushing close to her he offered her a smile. "Welcome to the Ashton Community. Maybe you and I could go out for a drink sometime. Get to know each other better." She'd backed as far away from him as she could in the confined space, then looked at him as if he was a worm on the ground.

"Go out with you? No way. Number one, I know you're a married man. Maybe that means nothing to you, but it means a lot to me. Number two," She'd looked him up and down. You're about 20 or 25 years older than me, closer to my parents' age. So, no thank you. I'll decline your offer. Thanks, but no thanks."

William had wanted to lash out and slap the smug smile off her pretty face. He still wanted to slap her and had to restrain himself from leaning over the desk to grab her. While he waited for her reply, he studied her. He was sure he had her this time with little or no defense.

"I treated my patient to the best of my ability. I did nothing wrong. Yes, Lara Scutterby died, and we don't know why. But it wasn't because of anything I did or didn't do. Someone knows what really happened to her and I intend to find out why she died."

"Keep your nose out of it. The autopsy report and the toxicology reports should be back soon. Until we know one way or another, Lara Scutterby isn't any of your business. Her father wants you to be fired immediately. I, of course told him that as soon as we get the reports back and find out you are the one responsible for his daughter's death, Ashton Community Hospital will terminate your employment. I will then personally contact the Nursing Board with a full report and a request that your license to practice be revoked."

"Let's just wait for the reports, shall we? I followed all the protocols for treating Lara. There was no indication that she was at risk for sudden death. If you bothered looking over the nurses' notes and doctor's notes from the emergency room for that night, you would know that. There was a Physician's Assistant in attendance the entire time Lara was there. As soon as I saw she was in cardiac arrest I called for the Code Team. When they arrived, I stepped back and let them take over. That's their job and they're good at it. I took care of her to the best of my ability I'm sorry she died, but that wasn't my fault. Now, if you'll excuse me, I have patients to attend to."

"I'll be waiting for those reports, Ms. Williams. I hope for your sake that patient died from natural causes or Leo Scutterby and I are coming for your job."

"You do that *Mr. Mager.*"

He hated the way she spit out his name as if she had a mouthful of dirt.

"Just remember one thing when you come after me. You might cost Ashton Community Hospital their top Orthopedic surgeon. You know the Chief of Surgery? In case you've forgotten his name is Jerome Williams. My father."

She stomped out, slamming the door behind her. William did the only thing he could. He hurled the folder at the closed door in impotent fury.

Chapter Six

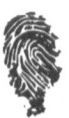

"**I** can't believe that Bas—piece of scum, Bully Bill. He threatened my job and my nursing license. I can understand Leo Scutterby saying things like that. Lara was his daughter. He was upset, she had just died. But there is no excuse for Bully Bill. He's had it in for me since shortly after I started working here."

Margarite grinned at Janessa. "You should have gone out with him. He wouldn't be all over you now for the least little thing."

"As if. Even if he wasn't married, over 20 years older than me and looked like a warthog, I still wouldn't go out with him."

Margarite's laugh echoed around the nurse's station. "Do you even know what warthogs look like? So, what did you say to him?"

It was Janessa's turn to grin, "The only thing I could. He knew what I was going to say before the words even left my mouth. I threatened him with Jerome Williams."

"Oh boy. I wish I could have been there to see the look on Bully's face."

"It wasn't pretty, that's for sure. Let's talk about something else. The man gives me the creeps and makes my blood boil. What about you? Any plans for the weekend?"

"Family. My niece, Daniella, has a softball tournament. You?"

"Not much," Janessa said. I'm just glad it's the weekend so I can relax. Mom and Dad invited me over for dinner tomorrow night. I'm glad they live only a half hour away. I'm not up for a long drive over the weekend." She began walking to the nurse's desk. "Now, we'd better finish up. The next shift will be here before we know it and we need to get ready for Huddle."

"Will you tell your father about Bully Bill's threat?'

"I haven't decided. Dad's used to HR's complaints about me. This is a little different though. They're threatening to take away my career and my reputation. He won't stand for that. I'm going to ask him not to do anything until we know for sure what's going on with the medical reports. We need to get ready for Huddle."

"Not much to tell them today. These two," Margarite motioned toward the patient's room, "It's been quiet and peaceful all day."

AFTER A QUIET WEEKEND of having dinner with her parents, lounging around her small two-bedroom ranch house and spending quality time with her Jack Russell terrier, Brutus, Janessa was ready for work and whatever surprises waited for her at the hospital on Monday. She'd dropped Brutus off at the doggie daycare, Nips & Yips. The place was clean, and the dogs well cared for, but the most important thing was that Brutus loved going there and spending time with his canine and human friends at Nips & Yips. Janessa could work her shift and not worry about her little buddy.

The tests and autopsy were still not back on Lara Scutterby; that would take more time. In the meantime, Janessa was in limbo. She was running out of options and people to question. So far, her questions had netted a big fat zero for information. But until the autopsy results came back, there was nothing else to do but keep her eyes and ears open and keep asking questions. No matter what Bully Bill said, she wasn't going to stop talking to anyone who might know something about Lara's death.

Janessa exited the elevator and made her way to the Critical Care unit. She and Margarite rode in separate cars today because they each had other commitments after work. Most days they rode together if they were both working in the Critical Care Unit and neither had a commitment after work. She wasn't surprised to see that Margarite hadn't made it to work yet. *No matter, there was still another few minutes before we have to be here for the change of shift Huddle.* It usually took about five minutes to get the patient reports from the previous shift.

Just as Janessa and the two nurses from the previous shift were about to begin, Margarite breezed in through the connecting doors. "Sorry I'm a little late. My car decided to act up this morning, but luckily Pete, my mechanic lives across the street. He had it running in a couple of minutes, so I was good to go in a short time."

Beth, one of the night nurses looked at her watch and smiled. "You're right on time. We were just about to begin. You're lucky your guy lives so close. I drive an hour to see my mechanic. And if the car won't start, the flatbed comes to haul it away. Hundreds of dollars later, I might get my car back."

"Peter and I have been friends and neighbors for years. He's actually a family friend. He and his wife are my parents' age. Growing up, we were in and out of their house as much as we were in our own. My folks don't see them as much since my parents moved to Connecticut."

"Connections like that are great." Beth said, a wistful look on her face. "Both of my parents passed within a year of each other. I'm an only child like my father was. My mother has a sister, but we haven't seen each other in years." She checked her watch again. "Good grief, I didn't mean to ramble on like that. Let's get this Huddle done."

Janessa and Margarite smiled at the night nurses, and a brief time later, those nurses were gone, and Janessa and Margarite were ready to begin their patient care. They had only one patient in the unit today, which made it easier to take turns for breaks. The other patient they'd had the day before went to Reese Memorial Medical Center over the weekend for more specialized treatment. *Makes it easier for me to go and question people, as long as I keep out of the way of the nurse manager.* Janessa pushed the thought around in her head but didn't say anything to her friend. "Hey, did you remember to clock in? Did you have time to do that?"

"Just. I swiped my badge and flew through the hall to get here."

"Great. We don't want Bully Bill to come after you. One of us is enough. 'The Amazon of Ashton' is here today so we have to be careful."

"Lovely, just what we need, Carla Potts in our faces. I'm sure you plan to continue sleuthing today, right? Getting around her will be tricky."

Janessa nodded. She certainly planned to sleuth. "I'll keep an eye out for her. By the way, how was your weekend? Did your niece win her games?"

"She was great. The girl has been playing since she was three. At 15 she is a total professional. She pitched in the first game, a no-hitter; she then played left field in the second game and made a couple of unbelievable catches. I have pictures to show you."

Janessa admired the pictures of the pretty young girl with black, curly hair in a pitcher's stance on the baseball mound. "Daniella is growing into a beautiful young lady." At Margarite's affirmative nod, she continued, "Does she look like her parents? I don't remember ever meeting them although I know they don't live too far away."

"She does, she looks just like my brother, her dad, Charlie. They live in Connecticut, not far from my parents, but it's far enough away that I don't see them very often. It's easier for me to go there to see them than it is for them to drag the three kids up here. Jason and Jared are twins. They're eleven. They play little league."

Janessa looked at her friend and frowned. "So, who in your family has red hair? Your parents? I know you have just the one sibling, and you just said his hair is dark like your niece." She noted the strange look on her friend's face.

"You're right. Charlie is my only sibling. Both of my parents also have dark hair. I don't know who has red hair in my family. I'm adopted, remember?"

"Oh nuts, I'm so sorry. That completely slipped my mind. I can't believe I made that careless remark."

Margarite laughed. "It's all good. I rarely think about it. I was an infant when the Barretts adopted me, so I've never known any other family. I've had a happy childhood. I know my parents, the Barretts, love me as much as I love them."

"I'm so happy I didn't offend you. My mouth gets ahead of my brain sometimes. I remember you told me a long time ago that you were adopted when you were a baby." An idea formed in Janessa's mind about Lara Scutterby and her father, but she dismissed it as impossible. She pushed it to the back of her thoughts to examine later.

Chapter Seven

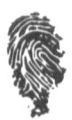

Janessa entered the nurse's station in the Emergency Room. No one was at the desk, so she listened for voices. Someone had to be around. Less than a minute later, the PA, Darryl Mintz, came into the room.

"Hi, Janessa. No patients in the unit today?"

"Yes, we have one and he's stable. Margarite is up there minding the place. I was hoping to see you. If you don't mind, I'd like to ask you some questions."

"Me? I plead not guilty to whatever it is." He laughed, a deep, hearty laugh genuinely enjoying his wittiness.

Janessa smiled at the big, dark man. He stood about six feet four inches, probably weighed about 220 pounds and was one of the gentlest souls Janessa had ever worked with. She'd seen his big hands move over a tiny 10-pound baby while cooing to keep it calm. She could trust whatever he had to say was the truth in any situation.

"I wanted to ask you about Lara Scutterby." His brows arched, but he said nothing. "Have you heard anything more about her death? When he shook his head, she continued. "Don't you think it's odd that a seemingly healthy young female just dies? I know young people can have underlying issues like heart disease, but there was no evidence of that with Lara."

"I know what you're getting at. We don't have any proof that her death was from anything but natural causes. True, when I examined her, I didn't see any major health problems, but I can't rule out that she had a heart arrythmia that we didn't detect, and it might have led to a spontaneous cardiac arrest."

Janessa sighed, "I know we can't prove it yet, but I think there's something peculiar about Lara's death. Someone did something to her. I can feel it."

"Is that why you're digging into this?"

Janessa looked at her hands then up into Darryl's handsome, dark brown face. "Yes. Something's wrong and I'm going to keep digging until I find out the truth."

When Darryl opened his mouth to say something else, Terry nearly ran into the nurse's station. She glared at Janessa. "What are you doing here? This isn't the Critical Care Unit. Go back there and let us get back to our work. If you're still on the kick about Lara's murder, forget it. No one here knows anything and we're too busy to listen to your stupid questions. Go back to your own job and leave us alone."

The hostility emanating from Terry was like a bitter taste in the air. Janessa stepped back in case the other nurse decided to get physical, although she doubted that Darryl would let anything happen to her. For the span of a heartbeat, Janessa couldn't say a word. She stared at Terry as if she'd never seen her before.

Terry seemed to be having a difficult day and was taking it out on her. Or at least that's what Janessa hoped was wrong. "I'm sorry. Something isn't right with Lara's death. I wanted..."

"I know what you want. You want to blame one of us for your mistakes. Lara Scutterby died on your watch, not ours. You were her nurse, not me and not Darryl. Now get lost!"

Janessa shrugged and half smiled at Darryl, then left the Emergency Department. As she went through the sliding doors to the main part of the hospital, someone called her name. She turned to see Marcia Connor who worked in housekeeping. The soft-spoken woman was mentally slow, but she was an excellent worker. Every unit she cleaned was spotless. Unlike many of the other employees at the hospital, Janessa was always kind to the woman. She liked her and noted that Marcia always tried to do her best.

"Janessa, I found something. I wanted to give it to you not that other one." She nodded her head toward the ER. "Terry?"

"Yeah, she's mean to me. She's not like you."

Janessa smiled at Marcia. The housekeeper was about four feet tall and was quite heavy. Despite her weight she was able to work and move around the hospital better than a lot of the other housekeepers.

"What did you find, Marcia?"

"I found these. I know they wasn't supposed to be where I found them, so I took them out and kept them to give to you. I knew you would know what to do with them."

In her palm, Marcia held two glass vials. Janessa pulled a pair of gloves from her pocket before reaching for the vials. "I'm glad you're wearing gloves, Marcia."

"Oh yes. The bottles were in the garbage can. I'd never put my hands in there without gloves. Only reason I reached in was 'cause I spotted them bottles. That wasn't the place for them."

"Where did you find them?"

"The trash can in the porter's closet."

Janessa took them from Marcia. Two empty 10 ml vials of Humalog Insulin, a synthetic version of the insulin found in the human body, rolled into her hand. The main ingredient in Humalog is lispro, a rapid acting insulin. These drugs treated type I or type II diabetics. This particular Humalog was a mix containing lispro protamine, which was a longer acting insulin as well as the fast-acting lispro. The insulin would get into the person's system rapidly to lower the blood sugar, then it would linger anywhere from two to four hours. Her breath caught. She wondered why they were in that trash can and who had put them there. Bottles like this had a special container designated for their disposal. The idea that popped into her head was too horrible to contemplate. *Is this what killed Lara Scutterby? How can I find out?*

"Marcia, you did the right thing by giving these to me. Does anyone else know about this?"

"No Janessa, just you. I don't trust no one else. You'll take care of it, right?"

"Don't worry about it. I'll take care of everything. Thank you again for doing such an excellent job, Marcia. I appreciate it."

Janessa raced for the elevator and jabbed the button for her floor with a gloved finger. She kept her hands in her pocket with the gloves on until she could get to her unit and get a bag to put the vials in. Maybe there were fingerprints, and she didn't want to mess them up. She could have kissed Marcia when she saw the housekeeper with gloves on. When the elevator stopped, instead of going directly to the nurse's station, she went into the clean utility room to find a suitable container for the vials. On one shelf was a stack of specimen containers. Inside the packaging was a small, clean plastic bag. Ripping open one of the packages, she dropped the vials inside the plastic bag and sealed it. *I'll have to give Frank Scott a call and ask him about death by Insulin overdose. I'm not sure that's even possible.*

Janessa left the utility room. "Margarite," Janessa called to her co-worker when she arrived back at the nurse's station. The plastic bag in her pocket felt heavy with the little bottles clinking together. "Wait until you see what I have."

Chapter Eight

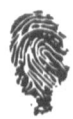

"I hope it's something interesting. Our patient was just discharged, and I've been bored to tears sitting here waiting for you."

"As you know, I went to the Emergency Department and started talking to Darryl. I got nowhere because he doesn't think Lara's death was anything but natural. Before I could go into it and ask more questions, Terry came in. Boy, talk about hostile. She practically shoved me out the door. For a few minutes I thought she was going to hit me."

"What's her problem? I thought the two of you got along very well."

"I thought so too, but she's been acting weird the last couple of times I went to the ED."

"And?" Margarite interrupted.

"As I was leaving, I ran into Marcia Connor, the housekeeper."

"Now you've got me." Margarite finished tapping the keys on her keyboard and turned to face Janessa. "You think Marcia killed Lara?"

"Good grief, no. It's what Marcia gave me that's so intriguing," Janessa pulled the plastic bag out of her pocket and showed Margarite the vials that were in the bag. "Marcia found these in a trash can in the porter's closet. The porter's closet that's connected to the Emergency Department."

"Holy sh...cow. Now we need to know who and why. Do you think our killer left these?"

"Possibly. I don't know. When I get home, I'm going to call Frank Scott."

"Why?"

"He's the medical examiner. I need to question him about insulin. I want to know if it will show up in the autopsy as a cause of death. We know that if it shows up on the toxicology screen it will be in amounts that would be normal to the body at the time of death. I want to know if there's a way to find out if it killed Lara. She wasn't a diabetic so if there's a way to detect an extraordinary amount of the insulin in her body, then it might be the thing that killed her. If there is then maybe we can find a trail to a killer and turn them into the police."

"Where's Detective Hottie? Why aren't the police investigating this death?"

"Leo Scutterby requested an autopsy; however, until the reports come back and point to a homicide, the police won't investigate it. So, we're stuck waiting and listening."

"The process takes so long that the killer has ample time to hide his or her tracks. It's crazy that we have to wait so long. Can't we speed things up?" Margarite asked.

Janessa sighed and looked at the bag in her hand. "Unfortunately, no. We have to wait, so, let's get ready for Huddle. I want to get out of here on time. I have a lot to do."

"This should be quick," Margarite said. "since we have no patients."

Janessa clicked on her computer and located her time screen. She scrolled down to the nursing schedule and spat out a curse.

"What's wrong?" Margarite asked, suddenly alarmed. Janessa rarely cursed.

"Potts! Look at your schedule and tell me if Potts messed with yours. She's got me working 7 pm-7 am Monday through Thursday of next week, then Saturday through Monday the following week. I won't be able to do anything but eat, sleep, and come to work. She's the worst manager ever. She has no right switching our schedules mid-month."

"Yup, she got me too. Damn. I start from 7 am to 7 pm on Monday. I'll only see you at Huddle. Oops, no I won't. I'm scheduled to work in the Emergency Department. To whom do we complain? Becca Doane won't do anything."

"Can't or won't. She's the damn Chief Nursing Officer. It might be a good thing if you can check things out and maybe get a little information while you're working Emergency. As for Potts, if I didn't know better, I'd say she's deliberately trying to split us up. Did you notice that Potts has hair similar to yours? It's a more faded red, and for a while I thought it was from a bottle, but I'm convinced that's her color."

An eye roll was Margarite's answer to Janessa's question about the hair. "If we're lucky, Potts will be the Shift Director next week. She either doesn't show up for her shift or sleeps through it. I should be able to sleuth with no one being the wiser."

"We all know Potts is in league with Bully Bill. I hope they don't think that will keep us from investigating. That's not going to happen. I know someone murdered Lara. We just need to find out who and why. If the tests come back, then we'd know. Oh well, we still have a few days before we have to do the three twelve-hour shifts and this weekend is free. The only problem is that by the fourth day when the twelves are over, you're too exhausted to move. Are you busy tomorrow? Maybe we can get together for lunch and go over the information we have. By then I should've been able to connect with Frank."

Carla Potts, a tall, heavy woman, had short faded red hair mixed with gray. Nicknamed "The Amazon" by the nursing staff, she tried to pretend that she was on top of things. The truth was that she was a terrible manager. The staff usually had no idea where she was or if she was even at the hospital when they were looking for her. When things didn't go her way, she was known to have a screaming fit at whoever was her target for the day. She would blame someone else for mistakes she made. Unfortunately, she was a crony of Bully Bill in HR.

"That is so true. You know she has her favorites, and we are not among them." Janessa snapped her fingers. "Hey, I just thought of something. Potts was Shift Director the night someone killed Lara. We searched and called for her, but she was a no show. I never did find out where she was. We dealt with the emergency without her."

"I'll bet she signed off on the sentinel event though, trying to put the blame on you so no one would look at her and see that she was derelict in her job. And..." Margarite paused and poked Janessa in her arm. "Would you want to be among the blessed few who bow at the feet of... *The Amazon*? She thinks she's intimidating because of her size, but I'm as tall as she is. Not as heavy, but I can hold my own. Anyway, tomorrow sounds like a plan. What time should I come over? Nothing is going on with the family this weekend so I'm free."

"Does 11:30 work for you?"

"Sure does. Here comes the next shift. We don't have much to tell them, so Huddle will be short. Murderer, here we come."

Chapter Nine

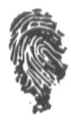

Janessa pulled her little Mini Cooper into her driveway. It had been a long week, and she was looking forward to relaxing with a glass of wine. But first things first. She got out of the car and opened the back door. Brutus, her Jack Russell Terrier sat patiently waiting for her to let him out of his seat. He hated the harness restraint, but he was used to it. He knew he couldn't roam the car while Janessa was driving, so other than the occasional sharp yip, he tended to watch out the window, getting excited and barking when he spotted another dog. Janessa wondered if they barked to each other about their confinement in their cars.

She smiled and undid the latches holding the dog in the seat. Brutus leapt into her arms and showered her face with wet doggy kisses. "I know, buddy, I know. The seat harness isn't the greatest, but I have to keep you safe." More wet doggy kisses followed. "I love you too." She glanced up to see her neighbor's curtain twitch back into place. "Nothing to see here, Gladys. Just a woman and her dog." She said it loud, hoping the nosy town gossip would hear her. She breathed a huge sigh of relief as soon as she unlocked her door and walked in. A glance at her watch told her it was after five o'clock. Frank Scott should still be in his office. He was usually there until after eight.

Janessa filled Brutus' food and water bowls, washed her hands then dialed Frank's number. He answered on the third ring.

"Medical Examiner's office, Frank Scott speaking."

"Hi Frank, it's Janessa Williams. I'm calling you about the Scutterby autopsy."

"I'm afraid I can't tell you much, confidentiality and all that. I have to give the final results to her father and the police in the next week or so. I won't have the toxicology screen back until several weeks after that."

"So, you found something?"

"Can't tell you that. You need to get the father's permission to get a copy of the report. Sorry. Rules is rules."

"It's okay. The reason I called is because I wanted you to check something. Does an insulin overdose show up on a tox screen or an autopsy? And how much would need to be injected to kill someone?"

"Probably wouldn't show other than the normal amounts we see at death. Postmortem blood glucose levels fluctuate arbitrarily. There can be an inconstant decrease in glucose after death, so hypoglycemia caused by an overdose of insulin can't be diagnosed accurately from a postmortem. A low blood sugar after death can be common. There are some random, expensive tests that I could run to see if that's a possibility, but I'd have to clear it with her next of kin. Frankly, I think the idea that someone killed her with insulin is a little far-fetched. What are you looking for anyway?"

"I'm not sure. It's just that someone found two multi-dose vials of two types of insulin. Someone tossed them into the trashcan in the porter's closet attached to the emergency department." There was a long silence on the phone. She thought she'd lost the connection. "Frank? Are you still there? Hello? Frank?"

"I'm here, I was thinking. Now I know why you asked those questions. Now it makes sense, but as I said, it's not likely she was accidentally overdosed with those drugs, but it's still a suspicious death until I can pin down an exact cause, but even if I do find it, you'll have to go through the family or the police to get any results."

"Thank you, Frank. May I call you again if I have more questions?"

"Anytime Janessa. I'm usually here until 9 o'clock except Sunday and Monday. If I don't take those two days off, the wife will have a fit. Especially now that we're empty nesters. We try to do something special on those days."

"That's good, Frank. Give Betty my best."

"Will do. Take care Janessa."

She hung up the phone after saying goodbye to Frank. Brutus was dancing around the floor then stopped to look at her. She grabbed his leash and clipped it on before heading to the back door. After Brutus finished his doggy business, Janessa decided to take a short walk around the town. She lived on the outskirts of Ashton so there was little need for a car except for work. The hospital was just far enough away that she needed to drive to get there. While she walked up the street, she mulled over her conversation with Frank Scott.

Several people waved or called out to her and Brutus while they were on their jaunt. She stopped at the Barkenaut, a pet restaurant in the center of the block, to get a treat for Brutus. It was fairly new. Their specialty was peanut butter dog treats, which Brutus loved and scarfed down in seconds.

As she resumed her walk, a police cruiser and an ambulance whizzed by, sirens blaring. Janessa stared after them, wondering who was ill. She pushed it to the back of her mind, knowing that she'd find out on her next shift, which thankfully wasn't until Monday. She resumed her walk until she realized that her stomach was grumbling. "Time to go home, Brutus. You had your snack, but I'm starving.

As much as Brutus loved his doggy daycare, he loved being home with Janessa more. He followed her around the house and watched every move she made. She checked that his water bowl was full then poured herself a glass of Pinot Grigio. As she sipped, she decided that a Caesar salad with leftover chicken sounded good. After the light supper, she and Brutus cuddled on the couch for a couple of hours before heading for bed. Brutus was a rescue dog Janessa had gotten two years ago. Someone left him in a kill shelter. Because he had a limp due to a slightly shorter back leg, the shelter was going to euthanize him. Janessa's friend Harriet, who worked at the shelter, called Janessa to tell her about Brutus. Harriet was on the verge of resigning from the shelter. She couldn't stand that they were a kill shelter. It tore her apart every time the shelter euthanized an animal.

Brutus was a happy and healthy little dog, and he was the joy of Janessa's life. He helped to calm her mind after seeing the suffering many patients went through. She'd become a nurse to help save lives. Finding out what happened to Lara was at the top of her list. If no one gave her an overdose of insulin, then there must be something else, something they'd missed. She felt a sense of urgency. If there was something traceable in Lara's body or body fluids, there might not be enough time to trace it. A killer might just walk free or kill someone else.

Chapter Ten

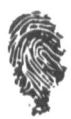

The next morning, Janessa was up early to finish her household chores. After she vacuumed, she tackled the bathroom, the job she detested the most. Good thing she lived alone so it wasn't too bad. She had shut the door so that Brutus couldn't come into the room. He had the disgusting habit of drinking out of the toilet bowl. She could hear him yipping outside the door. He sounded so outraged she couldn't help smiling.

While she cleaned, she thought about Lara Scutterby. She seemed so scared when she came into the hospital that evening weeks ago. That was why Janessa was going to do everything in her power to find out who killed the young woman. She had barely finished cleaning the bathroom when there was a knock on the door. A glance at her watch told her it was barely 10 am. *That can't be Margarite. It's too early.* She walked the few steps down the hall to the front door. Her house was small, so she'd been able to hear the loud knock even with the bathroom door closed. She pulled the curtain back and checked the side window of the door before opening it.

"Detective Halen, what can I do for you? Forgive me, where are my manners? Please, come in, Lance." As she closed the door behind him, Janessa caught a glimpse of her nosy neighbor Gladys Ketchum scurrying back into her house. No doubt she'd call the other neighborhood gossip, Patricia Lupid. By evening the two of them would swear that Janessa was in jail. In a town the size of Ashton everybody knew everyone else's business. Everyone in town knew the police force. There were two detectives, Lance Halen, and Tim Green.

There were also seven regular and three special officers as well as the chief, Greg Ivers.

Janessa motioned for the detective to take a seat on the slate gray sofa in her main living area. She hastily snatched up the blanket she and Brutus had cuddled under the night before. She looked around for her little dog then ran to the bathroom. "Be right back," she called over her shoulder. She'd forgotten to close the door. Sure enough, he had his little head and half his body buried in the toilet bowl.

"Brutus! Get out of there before you drown."

At Janessa's shout Detective Lance Halen ran into the hall leading to the bathroom. He gently moved her aside so that he could see what was happening. He erupted into laughter at the sight of Brutus buried in the toilet. Janessa elbowed him aside and scooped up the little dog. She glared at the detective before grabbing the towel she kept to wipe the dog after he did a toilet dive. That was getting to be a habit.

She glared at the detective. "I fail to see the humor Detective. He could drown."

"I'm sorry, Janessa, I mean Ms. Williams. You must admit it was funny seeing just his little butt and hind legs sticking up in the air."

Janessa had to smile. "You're right. He's so little it's the only way he can get to the water. He has to be halfway into the toilet. I usually keep the door closed because of his bad habit. That's also why I use only organic pet friendly cleaners. I was cleaning in there and must have forgotten to close the door when I heard you knock."

She walked back into the living room still clutching the little dog wrapped in a towel. He must have suddenly noticed the man and decided he didn't belong there. Brutus set off a series of barking yips while straining to get free of Janessa's arms to get to the strange man.

Janessa turned the dog to face her. "Really? Now you want to be a guard dog?" Brutus cocked his head to one side and looked at her. "Forget it. He's a policeman, so knock off the dramatics." Brutus settled onto her lap with one last half-hearted yip.

"Now that the drama is over, Detective, what can I do for you?"

Before he could answer there was another knock on the door. Janessa set Brutus on the floor with the admonition that he had to stay. He had heard the knock on the door, which set off a cacophony of barking. He ran in circles, but stayed where he was by Janessa's chair.

"Excuse me Detective, that must be my friend Margarite. I've been expecting her."

"I would come back another time when you're not so busy, but this can't wait."

Her eyes widened, and she stared at him for a moment before turning her back on him to answer the door.

"It took you long enough. What the heck were you doing. And why is there an unmarked police car here? It may be unmarked, but I know a p...oh."

The detective chose that moment to walk into the foyer. Margarite looked him over from the tips of his highly polished shoes to the wavy black hair on his head. That took a while, considering he stood about 6 feet 7 inches tall. She gave an audible gulp. "What's he doing here?" she asked in a stage whisper to Janessa.

"That's what I was about to find out. You're early."

"Yes, I figured you'd want to start our inves...oh." She subsided at Janessa's harsh look.

"Let's go sit in the living room and find out what he wants so I can stop wasting the detective's time. Can I offer anyone coffee?"

Her guests declined, and they all trooped back into the other room. Brutus had nearly shaken himself dry. He was so excited to see Margarite that he couldn't stand still. She picked him up and noticed the damp towel nearby. "Toilet adventures again, eh Brutus?"

"Okay, Detective Halen, can we finally get to the reason for your visit early on a Saturday morning?" She saw him glance at Margarite. "It's ok. Margarite can hear anything you say to me. She and I are close."

"All right then." He pulled a small pad and pen out of his jacket pocket. "I'd like to talk to you about Lara Scutterby, specifically, her death and the circumstances leading up to it."

"But none of the reports are back, are they? Do you have an autopsy report? A toxicology screen? I've checked and nothing is back. What is it that you're looking for?"

"The Ashton police department has been asked to look into her death as suspicious."

Margarite exploded out of the recliner she was sitting in. "What?"

Janessa held up her hand to stop her friend from saying anything else.

"I'm not sure I understand, Detective. With no reports back, her death could be from natural causes. Why are you questioning me?"

Janessa watched as a flush crept into his face. He looked down at his notepad then back at her. His gaze was sympathetic when he looked back at Janessa.

"You were the nurse of record the night she died. We're just trying to be proactive and make sure that it was a natural death."

"You just said it was suspicious. Whose idea was this? Whose idea was it to have you come here and interrogate me?"

"It's not an interrogation, Janessa please. That's why I came here instead of making you come to the station. Her father..."

"I see. That explains everything."

Chapter Eleven

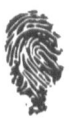

After the detective left, Janessa and Margarite eyed each other. Brutus had gotten bored and wandered off to sniff in the remote corners of the house. "What the heck was that all about?" Margarite asked as she headed toward the kitchen. Once there she filled the coffee maker with water and coffee grounds to brew a cup for her and Janessa.

"Leo Scutterby! I knew he would push to have the police involved. He thinks I killed his daughter and he'll use all his influence to get me fired and probably arrested for murder."

"He can't do that, can he?"

Janessa retrieved cups from a cupboard then went to the refrigerator for milk. Neither woman took sugar, so once the coffee brewed, each added a dollop of milk to her steaming cup of coffee and both were ready to sit down and collaborate about their findings.

"He can do anything he wants. After all, he is a powerful man in the town of Ashton. I won't be set up though. I agree with him that Lara was probably murdered, but the who and why escapes me for now."

"Okay," said Margarite after sipping her coffee. "What do you have so far? I tried, but I haven't learned anything."

"Me either, really. What we have is that Lara died abruptly within two hours of arriving at Ashton Community. Upon arrival, we did the standard tests. Her Vital signs were fairly stable although her blood pressure was slightly elevated. I started an IV, and per standard orders I gave her a bolus of Ringers Lactate solution. I drew blood for standard labs, CBC, chem profile, and those things. Then when the Physician's assistant arrived, he checked her out and ordered an EKG, which I did. He looked it over and thought it looked fine, but wanted to wait for the blood work to come back before he ordered any medications. She complained of pain in her right side, but, other than that, there was nothing. There was another patient in the adjoining cubicle and Terry was attending to her."

"Were you with Lara all the time?"

Janessa sipped her coffee and thought back over that night. It was over a month ago, but the images of what happened were clear in her mind. "I left the room briefly. I went out to the nurse's station and made some notes. Terry was in with her patient or at least I thought she was. I didn't see her come out of there until a little while later. When I went back to check on Lara she was unresponsive, so I called a code."

"And you said that when you were asking questions Terry was hostile?"

"Yes, but I'm not sure why." Janessa said, "We've worked together before with no problems. It was very odd. We also need to find out why the Insulin vials were in the Porter's closet trash. None of this makes sense and we have no idea if this relates to Lara's death."

"I'll do some sleuthing while I'm in the Emergency department. I'll let you know if Terry is receptive to me or hostile. I don't trust her very much. She looks like a killer."

Janessa laughed. "You can't tell a killer by their looks. She could be perfectly innocent. I'll admit some of her actions have been shady, but we can't accuse her of anything."

"Yet."

"What?" Janessa was trying to follow her friend's train of thought.

"Yet. We can't accuse her of anything yet. We need evidence."

"Margarite, be careful. We don't know who or what we're dealing with, so keep an eye out."

"I will. No one will suspect I'm sleuthing. Everyone knows you do it."

Janessa raised an eyebrow at her friend who sat at the table with a smirk on her face. "Excuse me? Everyone knows I sleuth. How do you figure that?"

"Cause, you've always been a "'Nosy Parker,'" not that it's a bad thing, mind you. No one will pay attention to what I'm doing. I kind of blend into the background."

"Sure, you do. Margarite, you have flame-red hair and you're 5'10" tall. You stand out wherever you go."

"Are you saying I'm an eyesore? At least you didn't announce my weight."

Janessa eyed her beautiful friend for a moment before answering. "I'm saying not only are you extremely tall and svelte for someone of your height, with gorgeous red hair, but you could also put a model to shame with your looks. So, no, you don't blend into the background, but I see what you mean. No one will suspect you of sleuthing and spying because you are so noticeable. You're also quieter than me. I tend to speak first and ask permission later."

"That's true. Now I need to go home and clean up before the weekend is over."

"Oh hey, did you see or hear the ambulance scream through town last night?"

"No, I didn't. I wonder who it was. We'll find out on Monday. I hope they're okay, but it doesn't sound good. The ambulance was on full earsplitting, siren blasting transport mode."

A short time later Margarite was gone, and Janessa finished the rest of the housework she'd neglected when her company was there. She decided to take Brutus for a short walk. The days were getting shorter and already cooler. She pulled on a light jacket and clipped Brutus' leash. The little dog danced with excitement as soon as he spotted the leash. He loved his walks. *Good thing he's small.* Vanessa closed and locked her door. *He's so excited he'll be walking me instead of the other way around.*

Janessa walked the short distance through the town, promising Brutus one of his favorite treats on the way back. They continued past the storefronts and down the lane where the houses thinned out then stopped altogether. Realizing the sun had gone down and it was now officially dark, Janessa turned to retrace her steps back into town. Out of nowhere, she heard the dull roar of a car. She had no idea of the model since she wasn't that into cars, unlike Margarite who seemed to store that useless knowledge in her brain.

Janessa made sure Brutus walked on the inside away from the street, near the ditch they were passing. A trickle of water ran down into a culvert leaving the ditch muddy and slick. The car was coming up fast, too fast, above the speed limit. It was almost on her when she turned to look. The car sped straight at her. She waved her arm to get the driver's attention, but the car kept coming at her. *That car isn't going to slow down or stop.* She grabbed Brutus and jumped into the ditch at the side of the road. Instead of stopping the driver gunned the engine and sped off in the direction of town.

Everything happened so fast that she didn't have time to see the color of the car, the license plate, or any distinguishing marks. The lights, on high beam, had blinded her. Bruised and covered in mud she pulled herself and Brutus, who'd started to whimper, out of the ditch and made her way home listening for sounds that the car was returning. When she heard nothing, she hurried home with a shivering, whimpering dog in her arms. After she'd given herself and Brutus a bath, prepared a quick meal and fed them both, they settled on the couch in front of the television to watch re-runs of Law and Order before heading to bed.

Chapter Twelve

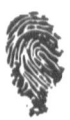

"Janessa, you'll never guess who was in that ambulance the other night?"

"What? Margarite, what time is it?" Janessa asked, fumbling for her watch, which she'd placed on her nightstand. Looking at the time, she saw that she still had about two hours before she had to be ready for work. "This better be good. I was sound asleep."

"Leo Scutterby! He had a heart attack. He's in the Critical Care Unit."

Janessa, fully awake now swung her legs to the side of the bed and sat upright. "What? Leo is in the Unit? Is he okay? I wonder what this will do to the investigation. Thank God he's not in the Emergency Department. We might lose him too."

"You've got that right. They said the attack was mild and that he'll be discharged in a couple of days. They've already scheduled him for cardiac rehab."

"Wow. It's even more important that we find out what happened to Lara. It's also important that someone watches Leo, while he's in there so that nothing happens to him. Has Terry been around him? I don't really trust her."

"That's the weird thing, she's been calling the Unit and asking how he is doing. I swear I saw her crying shortly after they admitted him to the Critical Care Unit. Something's up with her."

"That is odd. I didn't think she even really knew the man. Why is she so concerned about him? The weirder she acts, the more I think she's connected to Lara's death, but I have no way of proving it."

"She's not the only one. Potts has been hovering as well."

"That's no surprise. Potts hovers over every VIP trying to curry favor with them. If he's smart, he'll tell her to get lost. She's a real piece of work. Thanks for giving me the heads up."

Later that evening, Janessa exited the elevator and walked through the double doors to the Critical Care Unit. She knew she was working with Melissa Truscott, which was good. Melissa was a good nurse, friendly, with a no-nonsense attitude. Janessa took a seat and listened intently at Huddle where she learned about the two patients in the Critical Care Unit.

"Mr. Lyons, in room 401, came in this morning with ischemic heart disease. He's been given meds for the pain and to relax the heart muscles. He is having a pacemaker put in tomorrow morning." Scarlet Jenkins looked at Janessa before continuing. "In room 402 is Mr. Scutterby, who came in over the weekend with a myocardial infarction. The cardiologist says it was a relatively mild heart attack. Mr. Scutterby will start cardiac rehab in a couple of days and the nutritionist has been in to see him.' Scarlet paused again, "The other thing is, Potts says you are not to go near him, Janessa. He's not to be upset and he's still ranting that you killed his daughter. She says she'll be checking to make sure you don't disturb him."

"What nonsense. I had nothing to do with his daughter's death. "Janessa could feel her cheeks heat up. "He doesn't have to worry about me taking care of him. I don't want to see him any more than he wants to see me. He's already threatened me."

"I feel sorry for him. He just lost his only daughter." Melissa frowned at Janessa.

Janessa turned to look at her fully. "I feel bad for him too, but I won't be bullied and harassed for something I didn't do. He's threatened my job, and I won't tolerate that. I..." Janessa stopped. She didn't want everyone to know that she was investigating Lara's death. People tended to spill secrets when they didn't know she was sleuthing. "Anyway, I won't go near him. I don't need any trouble, especially with

Potts or God forbid, Bully Bill in HR. Besides, it's not like he'd win 'Father of the Year' when he spent little time with his daughter."

When Huddle ended, Janessa quickly read the electronic medical record of her patient before she went to check on him. She checked his vital signs, blood pressure, pulse, and his heart rate, which appeared to be stable. "Good evening, my name is Janessa Williams and I'm your nurse for the next few hours. Are you ready for your procedure tomorrow, Mr. Lyons? You're not nervous, are you?"

He shifted uneasily in the bed. The man appeared small and shrunken in the white sheeted hospital bed with the cardiac monitors hooked up to his body, beeping in the background. His face was pale, and his hands shook as he adjusted his covers. Janessa knew from looking at his medical information that he was 68 years old, but he looked much older. It was apparent that the man was suffering.

"I'm a little nervous, Janessa. would you mind explaining the procedure to me again?"

"I'd be happy to do that. We don't want you to worry about anything." Janessa explained the procedure in simple terms, happy that she succeeded in calming the man's anxieties. When he was calm, she left the room. She settled behind the desk at the nurse's station. She made a couple of notes in the electronic record before looking at the patient monitors in front of her. Something was off with Mr. Scutterby's monitor. Janessa assumed that Melissa was in the room with him. Sometimes moving the patient around caused the monitors to go a little haywire because of their sensitivity.

The call light was on over his room, but Janessa wasn't concerned. She thought that Melissa might have forgotten to turn it off. Sometimes that happened when a nurse wanted to immediately tend to the patient's needs.

"Help, nurse, help me." The shout was coming from Leo Scutterby's room. Janessa looked around but didn't see the other nurse.

Where on earth is Melissa? I can't go into that room, but if he needs help and she's not there I don't have a choice, Janessa stood and looked around again. It wasn't like Melissa to disappear when she had a patient to care for. Against her better judgement Janessa walked into the room where Leo Scutterby was hanging half off the bed. He turned to look at her as she came into the room to help him.

"You! You're not my nurse. Where is she? You get out of here. Are you trying to kill me like you killed my daughter? GET OUT NOW!"

The man's face was purple. The veins in his neck distended. The more he shouted the worse he looked. Janessa terrified he'd have a stroke or another heart attack, quickly left the room and ran smack into Carla Potts. Apparently, she was the Shift Director tonight.

"What in the hell are you doing in Mr. Scutterby's room.? I left explicit instructions that you weren't to go near him."

"He was calling for a nurse and I couldn't find Melissa so I..."

"You've caused a problem as usual. Melissa, tend to your patient. He needs you. As for you," She turned to Janessa, "I'm not going to say this again, Stay out of this room. I'll be calling HR tomorrow. This is unaccept..."

"Carla, call a code! Mr. Scutterby is not responding."

Carla stood as if turned to stone, so Janessa called the code. She prayed this wasn't a repeat of his daughter's death. Especially since she was the last person in the man's room before he went into cardiac arrest. He was screaming at her just moments ago.

Chapter Thirteen

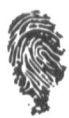

"What caused Mr. Scutterby's unresponsiveness?" Melissa sat next to Cardiologist Matt Trenton. She voiced aloud the question in everyone's mind.

"He had a cardiac arrhythmia that temporarily short-circuited his heart function. He should be fine with medication and if he's kept calm and without stress."

Carla Potts shot a pointed look at Janessa who studiously ignored her.

"But what caused the arrhythmia?" Janessa asked, biting her lip. She was afraid of his answer, but she had to know if she was at fault.

"Now that I've checked his bloodwork, I know what caused it. His potassium was dangerously low. I ordered potassium supplements after his initial intravenous dose. We'll monitor his bloodwork to make sure it doesn't happen again." His smile reassured Janessa that she had nothing to do with Leo's sudden bout of unresponsiveness.

"So emotional stress or emotional trauma had nothing to do with it?"

Janessa stared at Carla Potts, wishing her away. *Leave it to her to try to find a way to blame me for Scutterby's attack.*

"In rare instances that can happen, but I assure you in Mr. Scutterby's case there is a physical cause, not emotional. I understand that he recently lost his daughter. Losing a child does take its emotional toll. If it wasn't for his degree of heart block I would attribute his heart attack to the shock of his loss, however, I think it's a safe bet that poor life choices are the culprit. With time, medication, and cardiac rehab we should be able to get him back on track. He should have more good years."

Janessa breathed a quiet sigh of relief. At least she wouldn't have to face Bully Bill and possibly lose her job. At least not right away. She couldn't wait to get off this God-awful shift and get back to her days working with Margarite. Usually, she liked the relative quiet of the 7 pm to 7 am shift, but not with Potts hovering nearby watching her every move, waiting for her to slip up.

Thinking of Margarite reminded her that she hadn't told her about the car that nearly ran over her and Brutus. She'd have to keep her eyes and ears open until she and her friend could get together again. The identity of the car nagged at her. She should have recognized the car or the driver. What little she saw, had looked vaguely familiar, but her mind was blank.

The next night Janessa was on her way to Huddle after a restless day of little sleep. Nightmarish dreams had plagued her, and she kept waking up and looking at the clock thinking it was time to get up and go to work. She'd just drifted to sleep when her alarm went off. She could only hope it was a better night than the last one had been. She was up early so she took her time getting ready for work. She fed Brutus and filled his water bowl before she sat down to eat a bowl of oatmeal with a banana cut up on top.

It was evening, but working the odd shift, she felt that she was meant to eat oatmeal, which thankfully she liked. The drawback to working this shift was that unless Margarite could take him, Janessa had to leave Brutus alone. Luckily, her friend would come over later to pick up the dog. Janessa was comfortable leaving him for a couple of hours. She just had to make sure she closed all the doors, especially the bathroom door. When she finished, she patted Brutus on the head and left for her shift at Ashton Community Hospital.

She exited the elevator, walked through the double doors, and into a hailstorm. Leo Scutterby was standing in the door to his room with tubes hanging from various parts of his body. Carla Potts was nearby trying to placate him to no avail.

"I told you to get rid of that murderer. She just walked in the door so obviously, my wishes mean nothing. I'm a sick man and I don't want her anywhere near me. I'll have all your jobs if you don't do as I order. GET HER OUT OF HERE!"

Carla Potts glared at Janessa. "GO. You're working in Maternity tonight. Now, get off this Unit and do as I say."

"But I..."

"No buts. GO!"

Janessa fled back through the doors. She signed into Maternity and sat in a chair at the nurse's station for Huddle. There were no patients in Maternity. *What in the hell am I supposed to do for the next 8 hours?* Janessa smiled at the vacant-eyed nurse she was supposed to work with. "Okay, Barbara, what do we do with ourselves for the night? There are no patients. Are you expecting any deliveries?"

Barbara flipped through the papers in front of her. "We have nothing. Why are you here anyway? Don't you have any patients in the Critical Care Unit?"

"Oh yes, we have patients." A picture of Leo Scutterby flashed through her mind. "Another nurse was moved over from the Med/Surg unit to take over for me."

Barbara frowned. "Why?"

"Let's just say I have a conflict of interest with one of the patients. Believe me, I'm better off here. So is the patient."

"Is that Mr. Scutterby?"

Hmm, I underestimated Barbara, Janessa thought as she shifted uneasily in her chair. "You've got it. Mr. Scutterby and I don't exactly see eye to eye. So, Potts sent me over here so I couldn't do any further damage."

"Well, I'm happy about that. It's too quiet here when I'm alone. I mean someone comes to relieve me for breaks, usually Carla, but she doesn't really talk to me. She treats me like I'm invisible. I've tried to engage her in conversation, but it's no use. She hates me."

Janessa grinned. "She hates everyone. You're too quiet. I make waves. You know what they say about a squeaky wheel and all that. I just wish I could get to the bottom of the whole story of Lara Scutterby's death. Can I ask you a question?"

"Sure. I'll answer if I can."

"How did you know I had a problem with Scutterby. You're kind of isolated in Maternity. You're also working third shift. Not many people for you to gossip with. Not saying you gossip or anything like that."

Barbara reddened. "I um, might have eavesdropped on Carla and another nurse."

Janessa laughed aloud then leaned forward in her chair. "Okay, spill. What did Potts say?"

"She told Vivian Mann that you were nothing but a troublemaker. She said she couldn't wait to report you to HR. She hoped that he had enough dirt on you to finally fire you. I guess she's been reporting everything you do to HR. She's a spy for Bully Bill."

"I've always known she reported to him. The two of them are constantly looking for a way to get rid of me because I don't accept things as they are. I dig until I get to the truth of things, and I will find out the truth about Lara Scutterby's death. Someone killed her and I intend to find out who. I just hope I can keep my job long enough to do that. Personally, I think those two have a thing going on. "

Barbara gave her a wide-eyed stare. "Really? Potts and Bully? Do you really think so? I mean, she's always in his office. I don't really understand why she hates you. As for Mr. Scutterby, it's not like you're the one who killed his daughter. Right?

Chapter Fourteen

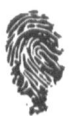

"It's so frustrating. I don't feel as if I'm any closer to solving this. I don't have any more information now than I did when I started." Janessa walked around her small house with her cell phone glued to her ear. She and Margarite had just come off opposite shifts. After the weekend they'd be back together on days.

"Did you get called into Bully Bill's office after the episode with Leo Scutterby?"

"Of course. Barbara, the nurse working in Maternity says she learned that Bill and Carla are in cahoots to get rid of me. One way or another, they want to get me out of Ashville Community. She overheard Carla talking to someone about me. After the shouting match with Scutterby Bully Bill called me into his office. He shouted, then Carla screeched and told me to get out of the unit. I shut Bill down very quickly. I told him that I'm not going anywhere and if he tried to oust me, I know certain things about him that he won't want to get out."

"That's not a surprise. I always knew he was a slimy creature. When I come over tomorrow, you'll have to tell me what you have on him. Then I can have the same leverage in case he comes after me. We'd better get our butts in gear and find out who the killer is, soon. Do you really know stuff about him?"

"No, but he doesn't know that. Speaking of killers, let me tell you about the car that tried to run over me and Brutus. We ended up in a ditch. Unfortunately, I..., Margarite, I have to go. I'll call you back. Frank Scott is trying to reach me."

Janessa clicked a button on her phone. "Hi, Frank, what's up?"

"I found something very interesting in Lara Scutterby's autopsy."

"Tell me, please. I'm not getting anywhere on my own."

"You did not hear this from me. The police already know, but my job is on the line by telling you what I found."

"I know. I'm sorry. I don't want to put you in an awkward position. I swear I won't tell anyone what you tell me except my partner."

"Partner?"

"Margarite Barrett. We're working together to find the killer. She's my best friend and we tell each other everything."

"That's right. I remember her. Beautiful redhead, right?"

"Yes. Now, tell me what you found."

"I don't know what you can do with this information because you still don't know who the killer is. I did other tests. I found an unusual amount of Potassium Chloride in Lara's heart blood. The level of potassium in the blood and vitreous humor was higher than the expected concentration after death. I've let the police know that my conclusion is final. Lara's death is a homicide by deliberate Potassium Chloride overdose."

"Wow! I didn't see that coming. I didn't think about Potassium Chloride, especially after housekeeping found the insulin vials. There were only a limited number of people with access to Potassium Chloride that night in the Emergency Department. Unfortunately, I'm one of them, so this doesn't rule me out. I was with Lara, and I was her nurse. I started her intravenous line and did the blood draws."

"I'm sorry. I wish I could give you something that would eliminate you from the picture. This just casts more suspicion on you."

"That's okay, Frank. You did your best. Now, Margarite and I will try to work faster than ever to pinpoint the killer before the police seriously come after me. Thanks to Lara's father screaming to everyone that I'm a murderer they already suspect me. My plan now is to find out who killed Lara and why."

"Good luck, Janessa. Keep me posted when you get to the bottom of this. My curiosity is piqued. I want to know who's bumping people off in Ashton Community Hospital using Potassium Chloride. I must admit the person was very clever using that. If you hadn't asked about digging deeper with your insulin theory, I might have dismissed the death as something natural like "dead in bed syndrome," which is more common in diabetics whose blood sugar drops too low during the night, but that's something you can pick up in an autopsy."

"I know, especially if you suspect undiagnosed diabetes, but Lara's bloodwork never showed that, and I suppose an insulin overdose would have shown up in a non-diabetic. Lara, however, was not a diabetic. I guess we can eliminate "dead in bed syndrome" in her case."

"True. And it just didn't warrant the expensive, extended tests I'd need to do to detect it. However, Potassium Chloride overdose is pretty easy to spot when you test the heart blood for substances like that on autopsy."

Janessa paced her living room and then stared out of her picture window. "Thanks anyway, Frank. I'll let you know as soon as I have anything to tell you."

Janessa hung up the phone and sat on the sofa trying to think of what her next move was going to be. She had to call Margarite and let her know about this latest development. It wasn't good. At least they now had a definitive cause of death, but no motive and no killer. *Time to research the Scutterby family history.* There has to be something or someone in the Scutterby background that had a grudge against Lara, or, against Leo and used Lara to lash out and hurt him. From the things Lara said that night in the Emergency Department it sounded like they had a rocky relationship. The woman didn't even want the hospital to notify him that she was in the hospital. By the time Darryl called him, it was too late. Lara was dead.

Everyone wanted to believe she died of natural causes, but Janessa had a feeling deep down that Lara's death wasn't natural. Before the coroner called her with the autopsy results, she knew Lara didn't die of natural causes. An unknown person murdered her. Someone injected her with a fatal dose of Potassium Chloride and Janessa was determined to find out who and, just as important, why. What kind of threat did Lara pose to this unknown person when she was in that hospital? Janessa grabbed her phone and dialed Margarite's number.

"Okay, what did Frank find?"

"Potassium Chloride. Fatal overdose."

"Good grief. We need to find this person fast. You know the cops are going to try and pin this on you. Did you have access to Potassium Chloride that night?"

"I know they will, and, yes, I could have accessed it, but I didn't. Can you come over tomorrow so we can work out our next move?"

"Of course. Give me time to give this apartment the once over then I'll be there. Oh, and Janessa? Do me a favor."

"Yes?"

"Be careful. This person has killed once. You're in the way of this person getting away with murder. Whoever tried to run you over with that car will be back. They're not finished with you yet. You're not dead!"

Chapter Fifteen

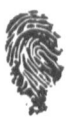

J anessa quickly finished her household chores including taking
Brutus out to do his business. She made a fresh pot of coffee and put
out cream. She was expecting Margarite any minute. She grabbed a pad
and pen and put them on the kitchen table as well. Time to get serious
and catch a killer before she ended up in a jail cell proclaiming her
innocence.

She heard a knock on the door and Margarite walked into the
kitchen. After petting Brutus, she pulled out a chair and sat at the
table. "This whole situation keeps getting worse, Janessa. What are we
going to do now? Potassium Chloride is on every crash cart, more than
enough for a fatal overdose. Every nurse or doctor or PA can access it.
It would be so easy to slip a drug out without having to sign for it. No
one would know it was gone unless they did an inventory of the cart."

"You've got that right, but according to what Frank said, even the
large amount on the cart was less than the amount found in Lara's body.
Whoever gave it to her had to get it from the AMD. The automated
system could supply the maximum, the crash cart could provide
enough to kill someone, but there wouldn't be the concentration Frank
found in Lara's heart blood. It's just a matter of time until the police
decide, along with a little help from Leo Scutterby, that I'm a murderer.
It doesn't matter that I didn't know the woman. I met her for the first
time the night she died."

"I know, but we need to hurry and find out who killed her. Did you
find out anything about the Scutterby's background?"

Janessa shuffled the papers she had placed on the table earlier. "A
little, but I'm not sure how helpful it will be. Leo is a widower of many

years. His wife died of cancer when Lara was 10. She had been sick for years before she passed. As far as I could tell he's a workaholic who didn't spend much time with his only child."

"So, the Scutterby's had no other children?"

"Not that I've found so far. It would be convenient if they had. We could just investigate a sibling who might have a grudge against Lara, but I can't find any other children in that family. Leo has an older brother who has no children. There has to be something. People generally aren't killed for no reason. Are they?"

"Not as far as I know. Think Janessa. Go back to that night and see if you can remember any little thing that might help."

"Okay. The secretary, Kylie Baker-Nichols said she heard the sliding doors open and close. We believe it was just before Lara was killed. She heard them again shortly after, but whoever it was went out, and disappeared by the time she was able to get up and look out of the door."

Margarite refilled her coffee cup. "Where were you when this was happening?"

"I think that's when I was at the nurse's station charting. I might have been talking to Darryl Mintz, the Physician's Assistant around that time. I remember that I had already logged in Lara's vital signs, started her IV, drawn blood and sent it off to the lab." Janessa stared absently as her friend added cream and three spoonsful of sugar to the coffee she'd just poured. "What are you doing? You never take sugar."

"Stress." Margarite took a sip of her coffee and grimaced. "Anything else?"

"Yes, her EKG. I had just taken an EKG and looked over the electrocardiogram because I had it ready for Darryl to read. At the time he didn't see anything of significance in the test."

Margarite peered at her friend. "Think, Janessa. Any little thing could be significant. What else did you do that night?"

"I was just thinking that Darryl didn't find anything significant in Lara's EKG. That means there couldn't have been anything given to her at that point. He wanted to hold off on any medications until the bloodwork came back. She was complaining of pain in her right chest, but he didn't want her medicated. He didn't want to mask any symptoms. He'd also ordered an x-ray, which was inconclusive."

"Where was Terry Meyers when all this was happening?"

"She had a patient in the next bay. I went to the nurse's station to chart, and I assumed she was tending to that patient. She was gone awhile, and shortly after that she came back and sat down with me. We chatted for a couple of minutes. Come to think of it, that was odd. Terry is not the chatty type. I went back in and found Lara unresponsive."

Janessa took a sip of her now tepid coffee and made a face. "Ugh. Cold coffee is even worse than putting sugar in it." She stood and walked over to the sink to pour it out. Before walking back to the table, she poured herself a fresh cup then sat back down.

"So, you can't account for Terry for a period of time. She could have slipped the Potassium Chloride in Lara's IV then pretended she'd been with her patient all along. There are two doors into that bay. She could be the killer."

"I thought of that too but there's one problem with that theory."

Margarite frowned. "What's that?"

"Why? What motive could Terry have to kill Lara. She knew her because she did make a couple of remarks about Lara being a frequent flyer in the Emergency Department. She also said that she thought that Lara wasn't a drug seeker so much as she was a Daddy attention seeker."

Margarite stared at Janessa as if she had two heads. "Don't you think that's an odd remark? Why would she say that? It sounds like she might have been jealous and resentful of Lara. I wonder why."

Janessa stroked Brutus's soft fur. She'd lifted him onto her lap. He was content to stay there and let her smooth her hand over his back.

"You know, I thought of that, too. There might be something to that, but how do we find out? I keep getting the eerie feeling that there's a connection between Terry and the Scutterby's, but I can't imagine what that could be. I think if we find that connection, we might just find a killer. I wish we had a way to dig deeper, but we're nurses not law enforcement."

Margarite's face lit up. "But we can dig deeper into their lives. My cousin Charlie Piper is a private Investigator. If he's not too busy with a case maybe he can help us."

"Oh my God. Is there any professional you don't have in your family?" Janessa laughed. "That would be so good if he could help us. I'm sure he has resources to get into places we can't. We need to get him onto this."

"True. I'll call him right away." Margarite pulled out her phone and started dialing. When her cousin answered she began to explain what was happening. They were interrupted minutes later by a knock on the door.

Janessa walked to the front door. Detective Lance Halen stood on her doorstep. Behind him, she spotted a police cruiser and a female officer. The lights weren't flashing, and there were no sirens, but the grim set to the detective's mouth told its own story.

"Janessa, I mean Ms. Williams, you need to come with us."

"Why? Am I under arrest?"

"Not at this time, but we'd like you to come to the station and answer some questions about the death of Lara Scutterby."

She listened to what he was saying but didn't for a minute believe she wouldn't be put in jail. "Can we do this here or may I drive myself?"

"Sorry, not this time. You need to come to the station. Officer Kristy will take you. I'll meet you down there."

"But wait, give me a minute to talk to my friend. I need to ask her to care for my dog. Do you have any idea of how long this will take?"

"I really can't say, Ms. Williams. It depends."

"Great. Hold on just a minute. Margarite!" Brutus shot out from beneath the table and started barking at Lance Halen. "Shhh. It's okay Brutus. You know Detective Halen." She scooped him up into her arms and felt his little body tremble. He must be sensing the tension she felt.

Margarite had come into the room behind Janessa. "Will you take Brutus with you? It seems I have to go to the station to talk to this nice detective. He'll need to go out, and if I'm not back, he has a meal of Kibble around five o'clock."

"Don't worry about a thing. Who else can I call for you?"

"Call James Crosby. My lawyer."

Chapter Sixteen

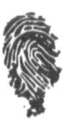

J anessa walked to the waiting police car, noting that her neighbor, Gladys Ketchum was looking out of her window. Within an hour, the entire neighborhood would know that the police took Janessa away with them. Shortly after, she walked into the police station accompanied by Officer Kristy who led her to a small windowless room. The stale air tickled her nose and dried her throat. The place was airless and taking a deep breath was difficult. There was a table with three chairs placed around it. A long mirror was along one wall. Janessa could see her reflection, but she knew the mirror was a two-way glass so that she could be observed by the detectives or any police who wanted to listen in during her interrogation. She eyed the metal bar that ran down the length of the table. With a shudder, she realized that it was to handcuff suspects in place so they couldn't attack the police or do other damage.

She heard the door lock click behind her and knew she wouldn't be free to leave the room until someone opened the door. Janessa had nothing to hide, but she was grateful she'd told Margarite to call her lawyer. Lara Scutterby's death was a tragedy; however, Janessa wasn't the cause. Someone administered a lethal dose of Potassium Chloride to the woman and Janessa wanted to find out who and why. She didn't do it. She just hoped she could convince the police of her innocence. She needed to get out of there so that she could continue her investigation.

Janessa had only a vague idea of who might be responsible, but it didn't add up. There was no obvious reason to kill Lara Scutterby. But someone did, and the police focused on her, Janessa Williams, when there was a real killer out there who might strike again and kill someone else. Lara's father was in the hospital and that made him a target. No one was listening to her suspicions so keeping him safe wasn't their priority. By keeping Janessa away from him everyone thought they were helping, but the further away from questioning him that she got, the less information she had. Without talking to him, she had a harder time finding the person who had killed Lara or figuring out why she was a target.

After an interminable amount of time, detective Lance Halen and another officer/detective came into the room. They sat across from Janessa in silence for several minutes. "Tell us what happened the night Lara Scutterby died." Lance Halen glanced at a folder in his hand. His voice was low, soft, and cajoling, the kind of voice that turned women's knees to liquid and had them begging him to take them to bed.

Not today. Janessa steeled herself against his charm and took a deep breath. "I was working in the emergency department the night Lara was brought into the hospital."

"That's not where you usually work, right? Why were you working in that department?"

Janessa cleared her throat and began again. "No. I usually work in the Critical Care Unit. Because the hospital is small several of the nurses are cross trained to work in other departments. The Unit had only one patient that night, so they only needed one nurse to care for the patient. The supervisor usually relieves us for breaks when there is only one nurse, so one person can do whatever is necessary with the patients. The emergency department was busy that night and they were short-staffed."

"Have you worked there before?"

"Yes, many times. I know the layout and the routine."

"You say you know the layout? Does that mean you know where and how to get the drugs that are there?"

"Of course. All the nurses know that. We have to in order to properly care for the patients."

Detective Halen looked at the folder again. The other detective in the room was silent. Janessa had never seen him before, and Detective Halen failed to introduce him. She studied his unsmiling face. He was probably in his early forties, older than Lance Halen whom Janessa knew was in his mid-thirties.

"How well did you know Lara Scutterby?"

"I didn't know her at all. The night she died was the first time I'd ever seen her."

"But you know her father, Leo Scutterby."

"Of course, everyone knows him. He's president of the board of Ashton Community Hospital."

"How well do you know Mr. Scutterby?"

"Not very well. The night his daughter died is the first time I've ever interacted with him. I've seen him at the hospital of course, but I'd never spoken to him until Lara died and he accused me of killing her."

"And did you? Kill her?"

Janessa looked over at the unnamed detective. She was horrified he'd asked her that question.

"Of course not! I had no reason to want her dead and I certainly didn't kill her. I just met her that night. She seemed nice."

"What about your co-workers? Do any of them have a grudge against Lara or her family?" Lance Halen leaned forward waiting for her answer.

"I couldn't tell you. I know most of the people who I worked with that night but not well enough to know if they were capable of murder. The patients were in and out of the emergency department pretty fast. We all had our own patients to tend to that night. If someone else needed help or their patient needed help, of course we all pitched in to do what we could."

"Tell us about the drugs. Who has access and where are they located?"

"There are a couple of ways to access the drugs. Both places are secure. We have an automated medication dispensing system that holds the drugs until it's time for the patients to have them. The other is the crash cart we use for emergencies and that's locked as well, but because they are for emergencies, they don't have a formal order from a doctor when we need them. Also, the lock on them opens easily for quick access. In an emergency, there's no time to waste fumbling with keys or conventional locks."

"What if you wanted to access a drug that hasn't been ordered?"

"If it's in our automated medication system the supervisor can override it and get a drug directly from the pharmacy."

"And the crash cart?"

"As I said, it has a simple lock and can be accessed by any nurse or doctor working in that area if they need emergency medications."

The unnamed detective made some notes, then looked over at Janessa. "Any nurse or doctor working in that area? Such as you?"

There was a knock on the door. James Crosby, Janessa's lawyer was led into the room by the desk sergeant. "Janessa, stop talking." James looked at the two men in the room. "Unless my client is under arrest, we're done here. She's a respected healthcare professional in the community and you shoved her in the back of a police car in front of her neighbors. It was humiliating to her and potentially damaging to her reputation. Unless you have a warrant for her arrest, next time you want to question her, you call me first, and I'll bring her here."

Chapter Seventeen

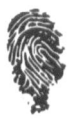

J anessa's lawyer dropped her off in front of her small house. She searched the bottom of her handbag until she found her keys. Before she could fit her key into the lock, the door opened. Margarite pulled her into an embrace. "I thought I'd never see you again. I waited for your call telling me the police decided to charge you with murder."

Janessa smiled and extricated herself from Margarite's tight grip. She'd been so anxious to get into the house that she hadn't noticed her friend's car in the driveway. "Not going to happen. They wanted to question me again about the night Lara died. They asked if I had any idea who would want her dead. When they finally figured out that I'd never met the woman before that night, they let me go. I can understand that they need to investigate everyone involved, but I wish they'd look for an actual killer. Someone is getting away with murder while they're wasting time trying to pin it on me. Pardon the pun but questioning me turned out to be a "dead end.""

"Not funny. I'm supposed to be the comedian of this duo."

At that moment Brutus realized Janessa was home and started whining and yipping. He danced around her ankles wanting her to pick him up. She glanced over her shoulder to see her neighbor, yank her curtain closed. Janessa pulled the door closed behind her and scooped up her sweet dog. He immediately covered her face with doggie kisses. "You'd think I'd been gone for a month instead of a couple of hours. Yes, Brutus, Mommy loves you too."

She turned to Margarite. "Thank you for watching him. I thought you were going to take him home with you?"

"He wouldn't go. I picked him up to take him to my car, but he cried and twisted his body so much I thought he would hurt himself. So, I brought him back inside and decided to stay here until you got back. I took him out back to do his business. I also put him on the leash and walked down to the Barkenaut. He really loves those peanut butter treats."

"I know. He loves them too much, so I have to limit him. Let's make tea. Police station coffee really is as bad as everyone says."

Janessa put Brutus down and began making the tea, while Margarite grabbed a chair and sat at the kitchen table. "So, what's next? We're kind of at a standstill in this investigation, aren't we?"

Janessa eyed her red-haired best friend. "Yes and no."

"What does that mean?"

"It means that yes, we seem to be at a standstill, but no this investigation isn't over. Someone had it in for Lara Scutterby and I intend to find out who and why." She went to her desk in the corner of the living room and pulled out her notebook. "Let's go over the facts again. Maybe something will spark a memory."

"Right. We need to look at who was in the Emergency Department that night and who could possibly have the motive to kill Lara."

Janessa scanned the people on her list. "Okay, we'll take it name by name and any relationship they might have had with Lara."

"We can eliminate you from the list immediately. No motive and you didn't know her. Who else is on there?"

"Darryl Mintz is next. He saw her briefly after she came in, but I was with him the entire time he was examining her. He also didn't seem familiar with her. If he'd met her before it didn't show in his manner toward her. Kylie Baker-Nichols was the receptionist that evening. She didn't come into the patient's cubicles. She did tell me that she thought she heard someone open the sliding doors to come in and then a short time later open them again to go out. She never saw anyone when she got up to check. Unfortunately, her desk is just enough to the side to obscure her view of the doors."

Margarite refilled her cup from the still-hot teapot wrapped in a hand-sewn cozy. "So, who's next? I know there had to be more people working there that night."

Janessa looked at her list again. "Well, the hospitalist, Dr. Trent was on, but he didn't make an appearance until I called the code. Darryl, the PA managed everything until that moment. Maria Connor, the housekeeper came through and emptied trash cans, but she didn't come into Lara's cubicle. I heard her cleaning the bathroom, but I doubt she knew Lara. Besides, I don't think she has the wherewith-all to commit a murder. She also doesn't have access to any drugs. This has to be someone who has access to the drug cart. She could never access the AMD for drugs either. I can take her off my list right now." Janessa drew a line through the housekeeper's name. She frowned at the next name on her list, Terry Meyers RN.

"What's wrong?" Margarite strained to see what Janessa was looking at in the notebook. Why are you frowning?

"Terry Meyers. She said she wasn't that familiar with Lara. However, she knew that Lara wasn't a drug seeker. She also said something odd. I didn't pay any attention to it at the time, but now that I think about it there might be some significance to it."

"What? Don't keep me in suspense, spill your guts woman!"

"When I asked about Lara's possible drug use, she said that Lara was a frequent flyer, but not for drugs. But that's not what struck me just now. She said something about Lara being a Daddy attention seeker. How would she know that unless she was familiar with Lara and her history? She would also have to know that Leo Scutterby was Lara's father. She was very judgmental. I wonder why and what she meant by that?"

"Ask her."

"Are you kidding? The last time I tried to question her she practically kicked me out of the Emergency Department. Then she reported to Bully Bill that I was harassing her. I had to go to HR and listen to him rant. That won't happen again. The lecherous old goat is just waiting for one more complaint against me so he can terminate my contract."

"I'll ask her."

"No, Margarite. If she killed Lara, we don't know why, and she could be dangerous. We'll just have to figure out another angle. It would help if I could talk to Leo without him screaming for me to get out of his sight and calling me a murderer."

"Okay. I won't go near Terry, but what if I talk to Leo? He doesn't really know me, and he probably doesn't know you and I are friends."

Janessa studied her friend for a minute. "That's true. You could see if Terry and Lara knew each other and what their relationship was if any. Enough for the day. Let me put Brutus out and when he's done, you and I can walk down to the Pizzarama and grab dinner. My treat because you took such good care of Brutus. We'll worry about Lara's murder later."

Chapter Eighteen

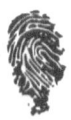

J anessa and Margarite sat at a table in Pizzarama. The pizza was thick with cheese, which was Janessa's favorite. She swallowed a bite of her pizza slice then looked over at her friend. "Hey, I keep forgetting to ask you about your search."

"My search?"

"Yeah. Weren't you going to go on one of those ancestry sites to see if you can get a lead on your birth family? Have you done that yet?"

Margarite's face turned bright red. "Not exactly."

"Why not? I thought you wanted to find your biological family and where you came from."

"I do, but it's not easy. What if I find them and they reject me again?"

Janessa realized her friend was afraid. "I'm so sorry, Margarite. I know this must be hard for you. But on the other hand, don't you think you might connect with family who's loved and missed you all these years?"

"I guess. I mean, I want to know who I am and where I came from, but it's ..."

"I know. It's scary. I'll be with you all the way. You won't be taking this journey alone."

"Thank you, Janessa. I knew I could count on you." Margarite reached into her purse and grabbed a tissue. After dabbing her eyes, she pulled a piece of paper from her bag. After straightening it out she handed it to Janessa. "We need to sign up for this. You never know what might happen. If we walk out of the hospital at night and security isn't available, we need to be able to protect ourselves."

Janessa scanned the flyer Margarite handed her. "Learn Self-Defense Tactics," the headline read. The course took place over six weeks on Thursdays from 7-9 PM at the Lark fitness center. It was a free course sponsored and taught by the Ashton Police Department. "We can do this provided Potts doesn't mess up our schedules again. She's such a piece of work. If she gets wind that we're doing this course, she'll deliberately schedule one or both of us for nights so we can't go. Let's just keep this between the two if us."

"True. We can't breathe a word of this to anyone. Most bosses would encourage us to go so we can learn self-defense. Not her. She'll do everything in her power to block us."

"Let the old witch try. You forget, I have a little pull at that hospital. I don't use the Daddy card often, but if Potts tries anything I'll let my father deal with her. He knows what she's like."

"True. Sometimes I forget that your father is the Chief of Surgery. Doctors of his caliber don't come along every day. Ashton Community Hospital needs him too much to make waves. I wonder if Detective Dreamy is teaching the class."

"Detective Halen? Hmm, that might be interesting."

Margarite giggled. "I bet he'd like to practice some moves on you."

Janessa did an eye roll. "I doubt that. I'm sure he has more important things to think about than me. I'm just the pain in the butt who keeps sticking her nose into police business."

"I've seen the way he looks at you. I don't think you're a pain to him. Maybe he'd like you to be more of a pain so he can see more of you."

Janessa threw a few dollars on the table for a tip. She had paid for the pizza when she ordered it. "Now I know you've gone off the deep end. Did I tell you about the other detective in the room with Halen when they interviewed me?"

Margarite stood and gathered her belongings that she'd placed on the chair next to her. "I don't think you did. Was he cute?"

"Not your type, honey. He was older. Very stern. He didn't speak much except to ask me if I killed Lara. He gave me the creeps. He mostly sat and stared at me while Detective Halen questioned me. I don't know what his issue was, but he definitely seemed to hate me on sight."

"Hate is a strong word. Distrust maybe. After all, you are a murder suspect. I'd be suspicious of you too if I didn't know you so well and know that you couldn't kill anyone."

Janessa lightly punched her friend in the arm as they exited the pizza restaurant. "Not funny." The two women walked back to Janessa's house in relative silence. When they got to the house, Janessa turned to look at Margarite. "I'll see you Monday. Let's hope there are no disasters, and the week is quiet."

"From your lips to God's ears. As soon as I get a chance I'll try to get to Leo Scutterby and question him. He doesn't know me so maybe I can get him to talk about Lara. Hopefully, he'll give us something more to go on in this investigation."

"Thanks. Just be careful. I don't want anything to happen to you."

"I'll be fine. You're the one who needs to be careful. The killer probably knows you're investigating and is out to eliminate you now. That near miss with the car worries me. I don't think it was just a crazy driver. Someone deliberately tried to run over you and poor Brutus. You should probably tell the police."

"You could be right that it was a deliberate attack, but I really have nothing to tell or show the police except for a muddy pair of pants. We both need to keep our eyes and ears open. This self-defense class might just come in handy."

The week was relatively quiet. When Thursday rolled around both women felt relieved. Because the fitness center was within walking distance of Janessa's house, Margarite left her car there so the women could walk to the class. When they got to the class it was full. The limit for the class was 25 and it looked like the class was maxed out. The instructor hadn't arrived yet. Janessa and Margarite slid into chairs and picked up the booklets that were on the chairs for the participants.

They had been waiting about five minutes when the door to the room opened. Before she could stop herself, Janessa let out an audible gasp. The detective, who'd been with Detective Halen during her interrogation, walked into the room.

He spotted Janessa and stared at her for the span of a heartbeat. His gaze took in the rest of the class. "Good evening, ladies and gentlemen. I'm Detective Pete Cranston. I've just joined the Ashton police department. Teaching self-defense is my specialty and I'll be your instructor for tonight and the next five weeks."

Chapter Nineteen

J anessa felt Margarite pull on her arm. "What's wrong? You look like you've seen a ghost."

"That detective. That's the one who was in the interrogation room with Detective Halen. He didn't say anything. He just stared then before they told me I was free to go he asked me if I killed Lara."

"Great! And we're stuck with him for the next six weeks. Why did we ever sign up for this class? Can we back out now?" Janessa watched her friend as she studied the detective. "I thought you said he was old?"

"No. I said he was older. We'll stick it out. But I'll bet you one thing. Teaching self-defense isn't the only reason he's here. I don't know why he's here in the Ashton police department, but it's for something other than this. I just hope he doesn't decide that I need to be in a jail cell before I can find Lara's killer."

"He's older, but kind of cute. Too bad I wasn't able to talk to Leo Scutterby though. He might have been able to give us insights into Lara's life. We might have been able to figure out who wanted her dead."

Janessa nodded. "We need to pay attention. I don't want to give this guy any excuse to look at me sideways. He scares me. He looks at me like I belong on America's Most wanted list. I'm a little surprised he's a local detective and not an FBI agent."

"Okay, ladies and gentlemen. My training partner is here so we'll start."

Janessa looked toward the front of the room. Detective Lance Halen was coming in the door.

"Oh, lovely. Just what I need. The two of them staring at me, wanting to grill me, and labeling me a murderer."

"Shh. Detective hunky wants to grill you a different way. Enjoy it. Let's hear what they have to say. We need to learn this stuff so we can be a little safer."

"As I said before I'm Detective Pete Cranston and this is my partner Detective Lance Halen. I'm sure many of you know Detective Halen since he's from this community. We want you to have a positive experience without fear. At the end of the six weeks, we expect that you will have the basic skills you need to protect yourself from an attacker. If you read the flyer we sent out, you will have seen that this is a very physical class, and that all of the classes are 90 minutes. We don't require physicals or anything like that, but if you have any medical issues that will prevent you from practicing the skills we're teaching, now is the time to let us know."

Margarite and Janessa eyed each other. As nurses, they were on their feet most of the day and although they weren't couch potatoes, neither woman was ready to run a marathon. They both felt the word exercise was a dirty word.

"At the beginning of every class, we'll start with warm-up exercises. Please move to the open area at the back of the room, but not onto the mats. We'll use them another time. Right now, we need to be on the hardwood floor for jumping jacks."

Several women groaned, but everyone moved to the designated area. "Catch me if I fall over," Margarite said. "Better yet I'll let Detective dreamy catch me."

Janessa chuckled. "Good luck with that. Shh. Here comes Cranston."

Detective Cranston positioned himself near Janessa and Margarite. "Ladies and gentlemen, let's move. Jumping jacks first, then we'll jog in place and after that we'll do squats. If you're not used to exercising be prepared to be a little uncomfortable for a day or two after class."

Janessa was jumping. So far so good. She was able to do it and she wasn't too winded after doing the jumping jacks. Margarite on the hand was a smoker so it wasn't long before she was puffing and trying to suck in air. "Are you okay?"

"I'm okay. Just not used to this activity." Margarite choked out. "I'm not quitting now."

"Okay, ladies and gents, take a breather, then we'll move on to jogging in place. Take it slow. We understand that you might not be used to this type of exercise."

Janessa noticed that he looked over at Margarite. Then he caught Janessa's eye. He didn't look at her so much as he stared at her. By the time he walked back to the front of the class, she was totally creeped out by him.

By the end of the class, almost all of the women and the couple of men in the class were like limp dishrags and that was just from the warmup. "Remember, self-defense is about awareness of your surroundings, being assertive when you're confronted by an adversary, and being able to use good verbal confrontation skills. We'll be teaching you safety strategies, and physical techniques that will help you to successfully escape, resist, and especially to survive a violent physical attack. One of the most important things you'll learn is communication skills that will help you get out of most situations. Next class, we'll talk about small devices that can help get you out of a tricky situation when communication fails. Good night, everyone. See you next week."

All of the women scooped up their handbags, notebooks, and other paraphernalia before heading out the door chattering excitedly. Margarite and Janessa were silent until they walked away from the fitness center. "Well, that was intense. Janessa said. "I just wish there were two other instructors though. Cranston makes me uncomfortable and Lance, well..."

"I thought you liked Detective Halen. Margarite stopped walking and stared at Janessa.

"I do. It's his partner, Detective Cranston that I can do without. He really thinks I could have killed Lara. The jerk doesn't even know me, but he looks at me like I'm a wanted criminal."

"Well, he did stare at you in class. Maybe he thinks you're pretty."

"I doubt that. He looks at me like he wants to handcuff me and throw me in the nearest cell. This class is going to tax my patience to the limits."

"At least you didn't have any trouble with those warmup exercises. They killed me."

Janessa laughed. "There are two reasons for that. One, I walk every day with Brutus, so I'm used to exercising above and beyond our job. And number two..."

"Don't tell me. I smoke. Okay, I'm going to quit, but it's not easy you know." Margarite resumed walking toward Janessa's house.

"I know it's not easy, however, we have a smoking cessation program at the hospital. You should check into it. It's free. I'd go with you, but I've never smoked so I can't relate."

"I know, and I will, Polly Perfect." Margarite cackled like a witch. "Right now, I just want us to get through this self-defense class so we can go and kick a killer's butt."

Chapter Twenty

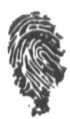

Days later, Margarite crept into the cardiac rehab gym after she ascertained that the nurse in charge of the unit had stepped away to use the restroom. Leo Scutterby had just started his workout. She and Janessa agreed that this was probably the perfect time to talk to him. He didn't know Margarite and if she was careful, he might open up to her about his daughter.

"Good morning, Mr. Scutterby. How are you feeling today?"

He smiled at her, then frowned. "How do you know who I am? Do I know you? Where's my regular nurse?"

"She's in the restroom. She'll be back in a moment. I'm Margarite Barrett. I usually work in the Critical Care Unit. I was there when you were a patient, although I wasn't one of the nurses who took care of you. Almost everyone in the hospital knows that you're president of the board of Ashton Community Hospital."

She could see him visibly relax. The last thing she wanted to do was cause him to have another heart attack. Margarite pretended to adjust the dials on the equipment. She knew there wasn't much time, so she decided to dive right into her questions. "I was really sorry to hear about your daughter Lara. I never met her, but I understand she was a sweet girl."

"Sweet girl? Huh. She wanted what she wanted when she wanted it. Yes, my late wife and I spoiled her so I guess I can blame myself that she turned out to be so selfish and self-centered. She was our only child and my wife doted on her. She gave her everything."

"So, you have no other children?"

She spotted the slight reddening of Leo's face. "No, Lara was the only one. Why?"

Margarite could feel the heat in her face and knew that she had turned red. "No reason. I just think it's a shame that you are all alone with no other children to comfort you now that your wife and Lara are both gone. That's kind of sad for you."

He laughed but not with humor. A harsh sound emitted from him, more cynical than sincere. "I don't need anyone else. I've been alone for a long time. Lara and I weren't close when she got older. Yes, it's a shame that someone killed her. She was too young to die, but I plan to make sure the nurse that killed her gets her just desserts. Neglectful bitch."

Margarite edged toward the door. She needed to get out of the room before he found out that she and Janessa were best friends. That would be a disaster. She wanted to ask him more questions but didn't know how to do it without raising his suspicions.

"Oh. I see. Do you think one of our nurses was responsible? I mean, we try to give patients the best care. Sometimes things happen that are beyond our control."

"Look, I don't know what business it is of yours, but I spoke to the police. I saw the autopsy report. Someone killed my daughter! Poisoned her! The only person near her at the time was that snooty nurse, Janessa Williams. I talked to another nurse who told me the Williams woman was always in trouble with Human Resources. She said that HR was looking for evidence of wrongdoing so they could kick her out. I intend to make sure that happens."

"What nurse was that?" She heard someone come into the room. "Well, ah, I need to get back to my unit, Mr. Scutterby. It was nice talking to you. Again, I'm sorry about your daughter, I..."

"Margarite, what are you doing here? Did you need me for something?"

Margarite turned to look at Janet Clarkson, the cardiac rehab nurse. *Oops, busted.* "No, I ah, just stopped in to see what brand treadmill you use in here. I'm taking a self-defense course and I wanted to exercise more for the class. We do warmup exercises that nearly killed me the other night. I figured using a treadmill would help."

"Are you taking the one with the police department? I've heard it's great, and free for us too. I wish I had time to take it. Maybe I can get in on the next round. So, hey, where's your partner in crime? I rarely see one of you without the other."

"Partner in cri...?" Margarite knew she had to beat a hasty retreat before Janet said Janessa's name. Leo would have a fit and possibly have another heart attack if he found out she was best friends with the *"neglectful bitch,"* he thought killed his daughter. "Janet, it was great talking to you, but I have to get back downstairs. The other nurse is alone, and my break is over. I hope you get better soon, Mr. Scutterby."

Margarite was out the door and standing in front of the elevator in a matter of seconds. She hoped that Janet would drop the subject and not mention to Leo Scutterby that Margarite and Janessa were best friends. She'd have to stay away from him for a while then test the waters another time to see if he knew anything. As she got on the elevator, she realized that he hadn't told her the name of the nurse he'd talked to about Janessa. Someone besides Leo was badmouthing her friend.

Janessa was waiting for her when she got off the elevator and entered the Critical Care Unit. "Well? Did you find out anything?"

"I found out that everything wasn't all sweetness and roses between Leo and his daughter. He said his wife doted on her and gave her everything. He says she was very spoiled. He also was adamant that they had no other children although his face got red when he said that. I think he might be lying and that there is another child somewhere."

At first Janessa was silent then she asked, "He and his wife had no other children?"

"That's what the man said. At one point his face got so red I thought he was going to have another heart attack or a stroke. He wanted to know why I was asking him so many questions about his daughter. I faked that one by saying that I thought it was so sad that he was alone."

"Whew. Good thing he doesn't know about our connection, or Bully Bill would call me into HR for sending you to talk to Leo."

Margarite sighed. "That was my choice, not yours. Janet Clarkson was the nurse today and she almost caught me. She asked why I was there. I fudged that by saying I wanted to look at the treadmill because I was thinking of getting one."

Janessa looked confused. "Treadmill?'

"Yes. I told her about the self-defense class warmup kicking my butt and that I thought walking on the treadmill might help."

"That was quick thinking. Hey, it might help. Now if we can get you off the cigarettes."

"You haven't heard all of it. I beat a hasty retreat when Janet started asked me where was my sidekick. I practically ran out of the room before she could say your name."

Janessa slumped in her chair and studied her friend. "Thank God."

"Also, apparently there's a nurse who has been badmouthing you to Leo. He really hates you and blames you for Lara's death. He says you're a 'neglectful bitch.'"

Chapter Twenty-One

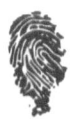

Janessa stared at her friend. "He said I'm a what?"

"A neglectful bitch."

Janessa stood up and paced the small, enclosed area of the Critical Care nurse's area. "I may be a bitch, but I've never been neglectful. I take good care of my patients and that includes Lara Scutterby. I don't know who killed her or why, but I'm more determined than ever to find out."

She sat back down and lowered her head into her hands and covered her face. "I can't believe this is happening. I have no leads on who could have wanted Lara dead, and the police are now taking a hard look at me." A vision of Detective Pete Cranston flashed through her mind. *He's taking more than a hard look. I wish I knew why.*

"So, what's next?" Margarite asked. Janessa noticed her friend's worried look. She wanted to reassure her and tell her everything would be okay, but she couldn't do that. She was fresh out of answers at the moment. The harder she tried, the more elusive the killer seemed.

"I wish I knew. We're running out of options and running out of time. If the police lock me up, I can't investigate. If I can't investigate then I'll be in jail for the rest of my life."

Margarite laid her hand on Janessa's hand. "That's not going to happen. We'll figure out whoever did this then Cranston will have to find someone else to target."

Janessa smiled at her friend. "You're right. We need to concentrate on the here and now and not speculate. You're a good friend. Thank you for sticking with me."

"We're more than friends. We're family and we stick together."

"True. Hey, have you done anything else with your DNA search? Any information on your birth family? Do you have any names?"

Janessa watched Margarite's face flush. "I kind of put it on the back burner. I've been busy wracking my brain about Lara's murder so much that I forgot about going any further into my birth family records. Besides, I need to talk to my parents first to see what information they have. I don't want to be chasing my tail and going in circles if they have useful information."

"Oh, Margarite. I know you're scared, but I'm sure whomever you came from, they must be good people. I never meant for you to put your life on hold to help me deal with this mess. Get back into your search so you can connect with your birth family."

"I will. Later."

"I'm so happy about that. I'm sure it will be an interesting journey. Wait! Later? Do me a favor and do it soon. I have a feeling something good will come from your search."

"As soon as we find Lara's killer, I'll get right on it."

Janessa tapped her friend's hand. "You're impossible. I'll make a deal with you. We'll do this together unless it drags on too long. If that happens, I want you to continue your search and let me continue this on my own."

"But I..."

"No buts, Margarite. Promise me."

"That's not fair, but I promise. Are you ready for tomorrow night?"

"Tomorrow night?"

Margarite laughed. "It's Thursday."

"Oh brother. That means I have to face Cranston's death stare. I wonder what his deal is. He's focusing on me, and I can't figure out why. I've never met the man, yet he looks at me like I'm evil incarnate."

Margarite shrugged. "I don't know what his problem is but look on the bright side. We get to hang out with Detective hottie. I think his issue with you is that you don't give him the time of day even though it's clear he wants to ask you out."

Janessa could feel the heat rise in her face. "Well, he kind of did ask me out."

"He did? When? What did you say?"

Janessa didn't speak while she thought back to the day Lance had asked her to go for coffee with him. She'd put him off, and he hadn't asked since. Maybe she'd completely turned him off because she was a murder suspect.

"Talk to me. What did you say to him? You refused, didn't you? Well?"

Janessa couldn't stop the smile that lifted the corners of her mouth. "Relax. I didn't exactly say no. He asked me out for coffee, but then we agreed that it might be better to wait until the investigation into Lara's death is over. It could compromise his role in the investigation if we started dating now."

"I guess that makes sense. But you are going to go out with him after, right?"

Janessa laughed. "Yes, provided I'm not in jail for a murder I didn't commit."

Margarite looked thoughtful. "Maybe I can go back to Cardiac Rehab to talk to Leo. I know there's something he's not telling us. He said that Lara was the only child he and his wife had, but what if he had a child with another woman? I mean, his affairs are legendary. We've talked about this before. We need to brainstorm and get further into Leo's life. I think if we find out what he's been up to we'll find the answers we need to solve Lara's murder."

"That might be why he and Lara weren't close. She didn't want us to call him the night she came into the Emergency Department. In fact, she wanted nothing to do with him, which was odd. Usually, when you're sick, you want your family near, but she didn't. There has to be a reason she was angry with him. She made it apparent to me that we weren't to call him. By the time someone called him, it was too late anyway. Lara was already dead. And, other than ranting and raving about someone killing his daughter, he was curiously emotionless."

Janessa registered the stare Margarite was directing her way. "What do you mean by emotionless? Didn't he cry or demand to see her?"

"Now that you mention it, no, he didn't. He stood in the hallway demanding to know why no one called him sooner. By the time someone called him it was too late. Lara was dead. Then he became more belligerent and demanded to know who had killed his daughter. We tried to reason with him, but he wasn't having any of that. It's odd now that I think of it, but the one who calmed him down was Terry Meyers."

"Terry? Did she know who he was?"

"Yes, she didn't *know* him, just who he was. I remember that she's the one who told me Lara's history. The other strange thing was that she said Lara wasn't a drug seeker, but that she was a daddy attention seeker. It's as if she knew the family dynamic."

"That is weird. Well, we'd better get ready for Huddle. Girl, you'd better also gird your loins for tomorrow night's class too. Janessa?"

Janessa looked up from the computer where she was making notes about the patient she'd taken care of that day. "Huh."

"I just thought of something terrible. Wouldn't it be strange if Cranston was related to Leo Scutterby and that's why he has it in for you?"

"Strange? No, that would be a catastrophe."

Chapter Twenty-Two

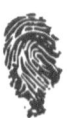

The next night Janessa and Margarite walked to the Lark Fitness Center for their self-defense class. Both women were anxious about the night ahead, but Janessa was especially apprehensive about how Detective Cranston would treat her. She thought it might be a conflict of interest if he was related to the Scutterbys and was working on Lara's case. However, she knew nothing about the human resources policies of the Ashton police department. Maybe it didn't matter to them if Cranston had a personal stake in the case.

Janessa and Margarite entered the fitness center and placed their jackets on the hooks in the hallway. The weather had turned cool. Fall was in the air, but by the time the women finished with their class they'd be hot and sweating. Janessa walked into the classroom first and looked around. She spotted Lance Halen talking to another student. He saw Janessa and smiled at her. Her smile faded as she caught a glimpse of Detective Cranston across the room. He glanced up and then continued to stare at Janessa.

Margarite poked her in the ribs. "Your new best friend is all about you already. The class hasn't even started. I really wish we could talk to him and find out what his problem is with you. Maybe I can get close to him and find out."

Janessa faced her friend. "Maybe you can."

Margarite stared at her as if she was crazy. "What are you talking about? Have you lost your mind? I can't talk to him."

Janessa smiled; her eyes held a cold, hard look. "I can't, but you can start a conversation with him when you ask for his help with a maneuver later in the class. Ask him where he's from, how long he's been a detective, and how he ended up in the Ashton PD. You know, stuff like that."

"Me! Why do I have to be the one to do that? I don't even know the man."

"Neither do I and I hardly think he'll make small talk with me, but you're a different story. I think he might open up to you. We need to find out if he's related to the Scutterbys. That's the only reason I can think of for his attitude toward me. There really isn't any other reason. There must be some kind of connection with that family. I don't want to stand and stare at him to see if I can detect a resemblance. But you might be able to get something from him."

"Why don't you ask Lance?" Margarite asked. Her face reddened. "I mean, what if he comes after me? He makes me uncomfortable."

Janessa stared at her. "How do you think I feel? He'd like nothing better than to put handcuffs on me and throw away the key. He gives me the creeps with his stares. I don't want to get Lance involved with this. Maybe I'm paranoid, but something is going on with Cranston."

"Don't look now, he's walking this way. We'd better take our seats."

The women moved to the chairs and sat down in the second row. They tried not to rush to the seats, but there was a sense of urgency to get away from Detective Cranston. Janessa forced herself to remain calm and walk to the chair. She wanted to run screaming from the room and not look back. However, it was important that they try to get all the information they could from Detective Cranston. Other than asking her if she'd killed Lara, he hadn't spoken to her. Why?

The class progressed and when Janessa ran into a problem with a technique, she caught Lance Halen's eye and signaled for him to come over. As he walked her way, out of the corner of her eye she spotted Cranston making a move toward her. Luckily, Margarite saw what was happening and called out to the detective. He turned toward her with a final glance at Janessa.

Lance showed her how to correct her stance to get the result she needed for the self-defense maneuver he showed her. When he walked away, she risked a glance at her friend and her "foe," detective Cranston. Janessa didn't know what Margarite said to him, but they were deep in conversation. She continued to watch as he showed Margarite a couple of moves involving her arms and swiveling her hips. She saw Margarite duplicate his actions, smile at him, and walk away. She noticed that he was smiling until he caught Janessa looking at him. The smile faded from his face. A scowl replaced it with an astonishing speed.

Janessa looked away and made her way back to her seat. Minutes later after the men lectured the students, the class was over. The two women made their way out of the classroom, down the hall, and out of the fitness building after grabbing their jackets. Janessa breathed a sigh of relief when she was away from Detective Cranston. She couldn't wait until she and Margarite were away from the building so she could find out if her friend had gotten any information from the man.

When the two women reached Janessa's house, she unlocked the door. They were immediately bombarded by Brutus. His little tail wagged furiously. He went from one woman to another trying to crawl up their legs he was so excited to see them. "Come on, Brutus. Outside boy. I'm sure you need a potty break."

Janessa opened the back door so that Brutus could go out and do his business. "As soon as I let him back in, we can talk, Margarite. Do you want a drink? Coffee, tea, wine? I even have beer if you want that."

"I'll switch it up and take a beer, thanks. I have so much to tell you."

"Grab one for me too, will you? I'm so nervous. I can't wait to hear what you found out, but I kind of dread it too. Come on, Brutus. You're done, big guy. There's nothing else for you to see out there." The little dog kept sniffing something in the corner of the backyard, ignoring Janessa. "Brutus! Treat boy, want a treat?" She went to the cupboard and took the top off the treat jar. Within seconds, Brutus ran into the house and skidded across the kitchen floor landing in front of Janessa.

She gave him a peanut butter doggie treat, then accepted the cold beer Margarite held out to her.

"Okay. I'm ready, what did you learn about my nemesis?"

"So much you wouldn't believe it. You won't believe who Pete Cranston is and why he joined the Ashville police department."

Janessa motioned for them to go into the living room and sit. "Should I be worried? I mean with the evil looks he gives me it wouldn't be a surprise to find out that he's a hitman disguised as a cop who wants to kill me." She saw Margarite's face turn red. "What? Is that it? He's out to kill me, isn't he?"

"Close. He's not a hitman, but he is out to get you."

Chapter Twenty-Three

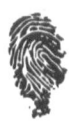

J anessa stared at Margarite. "Okay, give. Who is Cranston and what does he want with me?"

"I asked him why he moved here and joined the Ashville PD. He said a close relative had contacted him with a problem. So, he put in for a transfer to Ashville."

"Wait, where is he from? Who is the relative? What is their problem?"

"Whoa, one thing at a time. I started probing him about the relative, but he didn't answer. He started questioning me about you, but I shut him down."

"What did he want to know about me?"

Margarite shifted on the sofa and lowered her gaze. When she looked back at her, Janessa knew this was going to be bad. She was having a hard time reconciling that someone hated her that much for no reason. Perceived wrongdoing, but with no basis in fact. *I thought cops were all about truth and the facts.*

"He wanted to know if I'd ever witnessed you abusing your patients. When I asked him why he would make such a terrible accusation, he said he'd heard rumors about you. He said he wasn't accusing you, he just wanted to know because of these so-called rumors. I told him there was absolutely no truth to the rumors and that you were one of the best nurses I'd ever worked with. I also said that someone was trying to steer him in the wrong direction and away from whoever was the true murderer. I was furious and told him you've done nothing wrong, and that he needed to focus his attention elsewhere."

"Thank you, Margarite. You're a great, loyal friend."

"I spoke the truth. You would never hurt anyone."

At the sound of Margarite's voice, which had become elevated, Brutus put his paw on her knee as if to comfort her. Janessa watched her friend as she scooped him up and stroked his soft fur. "Brutus thinks you're upset. He's trying to comfort you."

"I know. He's a good friend, too. Loyal, as well."

"So, what else did Cranston have to say? Did you get any information about his background?"

"Not really, other than he came here at a relative's request. He dodged my questions and focused on you. I don't know if my conversation helped you or not. I walked away from him because I couldn't contain my fury at his line of questioning."

"Damn, I was hoping we'd learn more about him" She smiled at Margarite. "Apparently he's oblivious to your charm and beauty."

"He's oblivious, period. I didn't care for his attitude and the way he tried to twist whatever I said to him. He's very single-minded and focused on proving that you killed Lara. He didn't say it, but I'll bet you he's somehow connected to Leo Scutterby. I wish I could follow him to see what he's up to when he's off duty."

"Maybe we can." Margarite looked at her as if she had lost her mind.

"We can't do that. If we're caught, we'll be so screwed. Besides, we don't know diddly about checking into someone's background."

"We can't do it, but your cousin Charlie Piper can. He owes us anyway. He blew us off before but tell him this is a matter of life and death. He has to help us this time."

"Life and death?"

Janessa sighed and stared at her friend. "Yes, Margarite. If I have to spend the rest of my life in prison it will kill me. You have to convince Charlie to help us. I know he said he couldn't take on another case last time we asked him, but this really is an emergency. Call him and see if he can dig into Leo and Cranston's backgrounds. See if he can find a connection between the two men. There has to be something there."

"Great, I'm on it. I'll convince Charlie somehow. Worse comes to worst I'll threaten to tell his mother that he won't help me."

"How will that help us?"

She watched as Margarite's face scrunched into a frown. "You don't know his mother. Aunt Jezebel is hell-bent on keeping her family in line no matter what and no matter how old they are or where they live."

"Jezebel?"

"Yes. That's her real name too. It's how she keeps everyone in line. No one dares to laugh at her. She still hasn't forgiven her parents for that name. Thank God all of her kids have normal names, and she rules them with an iron fist."

Janessa laughed until she choked. "Hmm. Jezebel. But aren't all of her children adults? How can she still have such tight control?"

"Yes, her last son just graduated from college. So, tell me, would you want to argue with someone named Jezebel?"

"Not in this lifetime. In the first place, I'd have to keep a straight face when I thought about her name. Luckily, they get to call her Mom, so that's not as bad."

Margarite laughed. "You're right. One of these days I'll introduce you to her. We call her Aunt Jez, so you should be able to contain yourself as long as you don't think about her full name. If you laugh in her face after you're introduced, you'll beg Cranston to take you away. He'll be nothing compared to the wrath of Aunt Jez."

Janessa straightened up and stopped laughing. "Okay, you win. I'll keep that in mind. I'll keep thinking of Jez so that I don't mess up when I meet her. In the meantime, you need to call Charlie and convince him to help us."

"I'll call as soon as I can tomorrow. He's an early riser so I should be able to reach him before I go in to work. I won't say anything about Aunt Jez. Using her is a last resort."

Brutus jumped off Margarite's lap and made his way over to Janessa, who was sitting in the wing-backed armchair. She picked him up and held him close. "I hope he can help us. I could use all the ammunition I can get in this fight. It's an uphill battle and the only person who will listen to me so far is you. If I can get enough information about Cranston, I'll confront him and ask him directly about what he intends to do and why he would think I'm guilty of Lara's death with absolutely no evidence. I want to know if he's looking for the real killer."

"That you know of."

Janessa looked at her friend knowing the puzzlement showed on her face. "What?"

"No evidence that you know of at this moment."

"Since I didn't kill the woman, they don't have anything to use against me. If they did wouldn't Cranston have made sure of my arrest by now?"

Margarite looked concerned. "Probably, but that doesn't mean he's not digging and trying to build a case. With his attitude, I'd say he's probably made up his mind that you're a murderer. I'm sure he thinks it's only a matter of time until he can prove it and lock you away. If he's related to him, Leo's rich enough to make sure you go to jail, guilty or not."

Janessa shuddered. "No. I refuse to be a victim of misinformation, rumors, and speculation. Call Charlie so he can get on the case. The sooner we get answers the better. I know there is a connection between Cranston and Scutterby. That detective wants to put me in jail for something I didn't and wouldn't do."

Chapter Twenty-Four

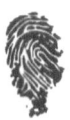

The next few days passed by in a rush for Janessa. At times she felt she was closing in on Lara's killer. Other times it felt like she was no closer than when she started. If something didn't give sooner rather than later, she'd be in a jail cell with no hope of proving her innocence. She wracked her brain and went over and over the events of the night Lara died, to no avail. Nothing struck her as unusual. She'd followed all the correct protocols, since she was a stickler for following the rules when it came to patient safety. She'd done all she could for Lara.

If only she could look around the emergency department again, maybe she'd see or remember something that would help her. Her chance came days later when two people called out sick, leaving the department short-staffed. The Critical Care unit wasn't busy, so Janessa would work in the emergency department until further notice.

In between treating patients, Janessa crept around the emergency department searching every nook and cranny for anything that might help prove that someone else murdered Lara. She still had no idea why someone would kill the woman but come hell or high water she planned to find out. Now that she had time and almost free range of the department, it was easier to search and listen. She could also question the people who had worked the night someone murdered Lara. She started with Kylie Baker- Nichols who had been the secretary on that night.

"Kylie, I hate to keep bugging you, but I wanted to go over the night Lara Scutterby died. Can you tell me again what you remember?"

"Why? That was quite a while ago. Why are you still asking questions about it? What was she to you? I really don't know much about her death."

"Kylie, I wouldn't ask, but the police have said that I'm their main suspect. It's confirmed that Lara's death was a homicide, and they think I did it. I tried to take care of Lara, but her father and now a detective in the Ashton police department think I killed a woman I'd just met. I have no idea what they think my motive might be for killing her."

"Sheesh. I'm sorry. I didn't realize. Sure, I can go over that night again with you. I remember most of it clearly. I couldn't believe it when I heard her death was a murder. That sure doesn't happen often in an emergency room. Do you have any idea who did it? Other than you, I mean. I know you wouldn't do anything like that."

"Thank you for the vote of confidence. Not yet. I'm still checking on things. Tell me what you saw or heard that evening."

Kylie went over the evening step by step, reiterating that she was sure she heard the sliding door open and then close not more than ten minutes later, but that she never saw anyone enter or leave the department.

Janessa frowned. It made sense that someone outside the hospital came in and killed Lara, but who? And why? From what she'd heard Lara was a nice woman and not likely to have any enemies. At least not any that would want her dead. "Is there anything else you can remember, Kylie? Any little detail could help."

"That's all, but I tell you," She looked around to make sure no one was listening. "Terry has been acting squirrely since that night. She's a little off all of the time anyway, but she's been worse than usual."

"Squirrely? What do you mean?"

"She walks around muttering to herself and she won't go near the cubicle where Lara died. If there's a patient there, she'll find someone else to take care of them. She also goes around telling the staff that they can't talk to anyone about Lara. She says it's patient confidentiality, but the woman is dead and that's not a secret. I don't think the HIPAA privacy laws apply in this situation. Especially when the police come around and question all of us about that night, or when they ask questions about you. I'm sorry, Janessa. I know you wouldn't hurt anyone."

"She told everyone they couldn't talk about the death. What is that about? This is very strange. As far as I know, she didn't even know the woman. Has she done anything like this before? Acted weird I mean?"

"Not that I've ever seen. She's always been little odd as I said before, but this time she's really gone psycho. I stay away from her whenever I can. I don't trust her. Did you ever think that she might be the one who killed Lara Scutterby?"

Janessa hesitated. She didn't want to throw out unfounded speculations about her co-workers. On the other hand, she thought the same thing in the beginning of her investigation. She hadn't changed her mind about that either. "I admit I had the same thought. The question is, why? If she didn't know Lara, why would she want to harm her? Terry is also a nurse and by all accounts a good and caring one. None of that makes sense. However, she did have the opportunity when I left the cubicle. Now I need to figure out what her motive would be."

The furrows between Kylie's brows had deepened. "How do you plan to do that? You're only in this department occasionally. Terry isn't even working today. As far as I know, she's not scheduled to be here until the day after tomorrow. Besides, there is no way she'll answer any of your questions. She's very defensive."

"You're probably right. Terry will never answer questions I ask her, so I haven't figured that out yet. I know I have to act fast. The police are hot on my tail, so I don't have a lot of time before they decide I'm guilty and arrest me."

"The police? Surely, they don't really think you had anything to do with the death?"

"I'm afraid they do. There's a detective who came to town shortly after the death. I think he's connected to Leo Scutterby, but I don't know how yet. He creeps me out and unfortunately, he's one of the instructors for my self-defense class."

"Wow! That could be a big problem for you. Self-defense?"

"Yes, Margarite Barrett and I are taking a class at the Lark Fitness Center. The instructors are two detectives, one of whom is Pete Cranston. He apparently wants to find me guilty of Lara's murder. He acts like he'd like nothing better than to lock me up forever."

"Can he do that? Lock you up I mean?" Kylie asked.

"Not unless he can prove that I've done something wrong, which I haven't. I followed all the rules the night the poor woman died. Her father is also hot to prove that I killed his daughter. He's pushing the police to come after me. I hope that DA Craggen dismisses the claims as nonsense, but you never know how things will go with the police. They follow their own agendas. And that..."

"*You!* What in the hell are *you* doing in my department?"

Terry Meyers stood by the desk, glaring at Janessa.

Chapter Twenty-Five

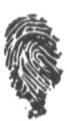

Janessa stared at Terry. "I don't know what your issue is with me, but I have every right to be here. The department was short-staffed, so the nursing supervisor sent me to work here. You're not a supervisor or Director of nurses. You have no right to question me, and this is not *your* department. I thought you were off for the next few days. What are *you* doing here?"

Terry's malevolent stare bored into Janessa's eyes. "That's my business. I'm here and that's all that matters. I'll have a talk with HR about you and your snooping."

Janessa straightened to her full height of five feet ten. "Go for it, although I know you did that already. You won't get anywhere with that strategy. I'm here to do a job. You on the other hand, have no business being here. You're off duty. I suggest you get whatever you came for and go home. And stay out of my business. You don't need to know what I'm doing or where I'm working."

"When I'm ready I'll leave. You have no right to tell me when to leave."

"Good grief, you sound like a petulant five-year-old. What in the hell is wrong with you, anyway? Go about your business Terry and stay out of my face."

Kylie was busy on the phone. Janessa didn't know if she was listening to the exchange between her and Terry, but she hoped so. She wanted a witness to the other woman's erratic behavior. Something was seriously wrong. She watched Terry unfurl her fists until her hands were straight at her sides. *She has real anger issues.* Janessa didn't shift her gaze away from Terry's face. She wasn't sure why there was so much misplaced anger at her.

"I hope you haven't been snooping around the emergency department like you usually do. I don't know what you think you'll find, but it's unsettling for everyone here, staff and patients."

"As you said, Terry, that is my business, not yours. Why does it concern you so much? Do you have something to hide?"

"I have nothing to hide." Terry turned and fled through the door to the nurse's station.

"Wow," Kylie said. "she really has it in for you. Why?"

Janessa didn't answer right away. An idea was spinning in her head, but she couldn't voice it yet, not until she had some kind of proof. Proof she could only get from Leo Scutterby or Margarite's PI relative. "I don't know what her problem is, but I intend to find out. Does she often come in and hang around on her days off? "

Kylie stared at Janessa for several long moments. "No, she doesn't usually come in like this. She's so hostile to you, I think she's here to watch you for some reason."

Chapter Twenty-Six

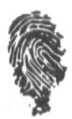

"I have to get to Leo Scutterby and talk to him. I have a feeling he's the key to all of this, including Lara's murder."

Margarite stared at her. "You don't think he killed his own daughter, do you?"

"Of course not, but I think he's the root cause of her death. For someone this was a way to get to Leo. Killing Lara was sending a message to him."

Janessa watched Margarite's eyes widen and could guess what she was thinking. "A message? Kind of a gruesome message don't you think? I mean killing his daughter was a hell of a way to get his notice. Besides, do you think he really cares that she's gone? It sounds to me like he didn't want to be around her and only in death is she now his beloved daughter."

"It certainly is a known fact that he and his daughter weren't close and that's why I have to get to Leo and talk to him. If I can pick his brains about his past and his life with his daughter, I might get to the root of the problem. However, I don't know how I can do it. He's made it clear that he doesn't want me anywhere near him."

Janessa stood and stretched. It was the weekend, and the two nurses were sitting at Janessa's kitchen table. Brutus trotted into the room, his water bowl dangling from his jaws. "Oh, my God! I am such a bad fur mommy. I've totally neglected you." She glanced at Margarite. "I'm glad he has a mind of his own and knows how to communicate with me." She laughed and walked to the sink to fill the water bowl. She turned to look at her friend. "Has your cousin found any more information about Detective Cranston?"

"Oh crap, yes. Charlie called and gave me a boatload of information. It totally went right out of my head. Apparently, Cranston is Leo's nephew."

"Nephew! I thought Leo was an only child."

"Well, he is, technically. He had a stepsister. She's dead now. Terrible car accident when her son was about five or six. His father raised him, but apparently, he and 'Uncle Leo' have stayed close. I imagine that Leo contacted someone and had Pete Cranston transferred here as soon as he found out Lara's death wasn't from natural causes. When I spoke to him, he said he was here at a 'relative's' request. But he wouldn't elaborate on that."

"No wonder he's been breathing down my neck. If Leo said I murdered Lara, he's here to prove it and make sure I go to jail. Lovely. Now I really need to talk to Leo."

"Have you thought about how you're going to do that? The man won't let you within 50 feet and I'm sure he'd be happy to call Cranston to arrest you for harassing him."

Janessa looked into the sink at Brutus' overflowing water bowl. "Damn." She dumped out the excess and set the bowl on the floor beside Brutus, who was dancing around in circles. I need to think about it some more. Something will come to me. In the meantime, just for a change of subject and to get off the death for a while, let's talk about something else. What have you done about getting your DNA results? Have you decided to do it?"

"Yesss, sort of. I've decided to go ahead and find out where I came from, but it's a big decision. It won't just affect me, but everyone else in the family too."

Janessa could hear the reluctance in her friend's voice. "Let me know if I can help, even if it's just for moral support. I know deep down you want to know about your ancestry, but I'm sure you're a little afraid of the results."

"I am and thank you. Until recently I'd never thought much about being adopted, but I'm getting older, and I would like to have information about, you know, diseases and stuff."

"Older? Well, I guess you're right. For most people, I guess it's natural to have information like that at our fingertips. When you're chosen by a family, you have to search elsewhere. It will be fine, Margarite. I have a good feeling about this, and I know you'll be happy with whatever you find out about your birth family."

"I hope I don't regret it. The secrecy about closed adoptions is what annoys me. Why can't they be open from the get-go? The child or children shouldn't have to search to reach out and get familial information. Like birth children, they should have access to biological information from the time they're old enough to understand about adoption."

"You have a point there. They should have access at an early age. Some adoptees do, but too many are kept in the dark and sometimes bad things happen because of it."

Margarite took a sip of coffee Janessa had made earlier. She set the cup down on the table and looked over at Janessa. "I agree. I'm lucky that I ended up in a great family, and I love them all dearly, but there's always a gap, a kind of hollow that you're missing something, and you don't know what."

Janessa stared at Margarite. "You're right. That gap or hollow could induce children to search for their birth families. I hope you have happy results, but not everyone does. In fact, they might find a father who left the family with nothing. Or a sibling they think cheated them out of everything they deserve, a sibling who has had all of the missing parent's love and in order to get that affection, they need to get that sibling out of the way. Permanently."

"What do you mean? Maybe I'm dense, but you lost me at a sibling's cheating them out of everything. Explain."

"I know we just said we'd get off the murder for a while, but this just popped into my head. What if the gossip was right and Leo had an affair early in his marriage to Lara's mother? What if there was a child from that affair? If that child never knew the father, then found out who he was later in life she would not only be furious with him for abandoning her and her mother, she'd be jealous of the sibling who'd had the father's attention for all the years she'd been without his presence in her life and his affection."

Margarite nodded. "You said she, so I assume you think the child is a female? Of course. It makes more sense now. Lara's death makes sense. If someone in the Emergency Department is that sibling, he or she could have gone into Lara's cubicle and killed her. I know you keep saying she, but it could just as easily have been a boy. Right?"

"Right. Now all I have to do is find out who Leo had an affair with and if there was a child. My bet is that not only was there a child but he/she works at Ashton Community Hospital, which would give them ready access to Lara. Margarite, we might just be on the trail of nabbing our killer. Thank you and your DNA."

Chapter Twenty-Seven

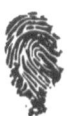

"Hey Margarite, I know I can't get next to Leo, but you can."

"Me? How can I get near him? I doubt he'll talk to me either. Besides, doesn't he know that you and I are friends? There's no way he'll tell me anything if he knows you and I are best friends. Neither one of us can get near him."

Janessa paced around the small kitchen. She straightened a tea towel she had draped over the handle of the oven door. "Listen, you talked to him when he was in cardiac rehab. Right?" She continued when Margarite nodded her head. "He kicked me out of his room and screamed his head off that I murdered his daughter. He never said a word to you, so I doubt that he knows we're friends."

"Well yeah, but I..."

"But nothing. All you have to find out is whether or not he had a liaison with another woman when he was married and if there was a child from that affair. Although I have to admit that he might not know about a child. Chances are because he was married, supposedly happily, he might have had the fling and then dropped the woman. If she got pregnant, chances are good that she never told Leo."

"And how do you propose I do that? I tried talking to him when he was in cardiac rehab and almost got busted then. I had to backpedal and beat a hasty retreat before he found out about our connection. We'd have both been in trouble.

"That was a while ago. He probably doesn't even remember you."

Margarite laughed. "I'm not that forgettable." She pulled at a few strands of her flame-colored hair. "With this hair, I tend to stand out in a crowd."

"Crap. I forgot about your 'beacon.'" Janessa smiled at her friend and reached out to touch her friend's bright red hair. "That's okay, we'll have to figure out something else. Maybe your cousin Charlie can do some more digging for us." She rubbed her chin, paced back and forth, then paused to look out the window. She turned back to face Margarite. "I wish we knew the name of the woman. That would make it so easy for Charlie to get the information we need."

"We know Leo Scutterby's name. Charlie's good. Maybe he can start there and do a deep dive into Leo's past."

"That would be great. Tell him this would have been early in Leo's marriage. So, it would be about 33 or 34 or years ago. I don't know if Lara was born when he had the affair so if Charlie can go back at least 35 years then maybe he'll find something."

"What about birth records from back then? If there was another baby born around that time, then maybe he could check birth records. Most will probably list both parents, but I doubt that any woman Leo had an affair with would do that. She may have put down that the father was unknown. So, there might not be a record that Leo is the father."

At first Margarite didn't speak. When she looked up Janessa could see the shadow of doubt in her eyes. "What if she went out of state? Maybe she had the baby elsewhere. How do we know where that baby was born?"

"We're so close to two other state borders we'll tell him to check the tri-state area. If that doesn't pan out, then we can extend into Vermont and New Hampshire. They're close enough.

Okay, so call Charlie and tell him everything we currently know about Leo Scutterby but tell him we need this information ASAP. The sooner the better. I have this feeling in the pit of my stomach that time is running out. Mainly for me."

Margarite laid her hand over her friend's. "Don't worry 'Nessa,' we'll get to the bottom of this. In the meantime, Leo can't stop me if I 'accidentally' run into him in the supermarket or the library or something like that. We both live in the town, so what can he say?"

Janessa laughed for the first time in a while. "What are you going to do, start interrogating him over the produce? Or better yet, how about the bakery? At least then you'll have some tasty treats to take the edge off."

The two women giggled at the thought of Margarite grabbing a baguette and whacking Leo with it to get his attention so she could quiz him about his past indiscretions. Minutes later a sobering thought came to Janessa. "The thing is, we have to watch out for Pete Cranston. I don't trust him not to manufacture a charge and throw one or both of us in jail. If you see him run in the opposite direction."

"You're right. I have no desire to go to jail. I don't plan to be anybody's b—-h! Well, you know what I mean. On the other hand, I think he's kind of cute. I almost liked talking to him the other night."

Janessa ignored her friend's last remark. "Let me know as soon as you've reached Charlie. Tell him it's extremely urgent that he gets any information he can as soon as possible. Now, I have to take Brutus out for a walk. Are you coming with us or going home?"

Margarite stood, then walked across the kitchen and placed her cup in the sink. "I'm going to head home. I have a ton of things to do as usual. Weekends are great, but they're over too soon."

"I'm with you there. I can never get ahead of everything."

Margarite laughed and pulled on her jacket. "What are you talking about? Your house is always immaculate. You love your dog. He's well fed, and you take good care of him. I won't say he's well-behaved. That's another story."

Brutus whined as if he knew what Margarite was saying about him. He danced around the kitchen and then ran to the door. He was ready to go for his walk. That was one word he understood. Food was the other.

"Where are you working next week? Are we together in the Critical Care Unit?"

"Not at the beginning of the week. I'm in the Emergency department again. Brenda Garcia is going out on maternity leave."

"You won't be there for her entire leave, will you?"

"Are you going to miss me?" Janessa smiled at Margarite. "No, this week I'll be there for three days. After that, who knows? I like working in that department. The downside is that I have to work with Terry Meyers and her behavior has been very erratic. She's made it obvious she doesn't want me there. Thank God she's not in charge of anything. I know she'd try to make trouble for me, which she already has. I'll bet she was the one who complained to HR that I was snooping in the ER."

"Be careful, will you? For all we know you could be working side by side with a killer."

Chapter Twenty-Eight

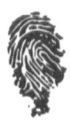

Later that day, when Janessa's phone rang, she saw that the caller was Margarite. "Miss me all ready?" She laughed.

"Hi, sweetie. Now, be serious. I called Charlie and he's on it. He says he'll get information to us as soon as he can. He has a couple of other cases he's working on, but he'll prioritize our case and start checking as soon as possible."

"Thanks, Margarite. The sooner the better. I can't help but feel that we're getting closer to the killer, but I also feel like the danger to us is stronger. By the way, we have a self-defense class this Thursday. You up for it?"

"Sure am. Maybe I can corner Pete Cranston and pick his brain. I don't know what I can get out of him, but it will be worth a try."

Janessa smiled. "I can't wait for Thursday. It might get interesting."

"Plus, you get to see Lance again. Up close and personal with him too."

Janessa laughed. "You're incorrigible. Yes, he's cute and he has asked me out for coffee, but until Lara's case is over, we can't really get near each other."

"Yeah, that sucks. However, if staying away from him means we catch whoever killed Lara, it will be worth it."

"I'm glad I have you as a partner, Margarite. There are times when you keep me grounded because you can be practical. Sometimes."

"And the rest of the time?"

"Let's not get into that. I'll see you Thursday. I'm working in the emergency department, so I won't see you until then. Maybe I'll find out some more information about our case. I'm not counting on it, but who knows? Maybe the killer will make a mistake and come after me. I'll be ready for him or her."

"Ready? How?"

"I know self-defense, remember?" Janessa said and grinned, knowing that Margarite couldn't see her.

"That's not funny. I don't think we've learned enough to defend ourselves against an attacker. Be careful. Just be a nurse, for once, and leave the sleuthing to the police." At Janessa's laugh, she continued. "I mean it, 'Nessa.'" I don't want to lose you to a killer with a grudge. Remember this person killed Lara with several medical professionals within arm's reach."

"You worry too much. Nothing will happen. I'll do my job and keep my ears and eyes open. See you Thursday."

After Margarite hung up, Janessa finished her chores before gathering everything she needed for work the next day. She was working in the Emergency Department, but for once it was a regular seven to three-shift for three days.

Once again, she was working with Terry, but the woman seemed calmer. She was actually friendly. Janessa thought about the other encounters when the woman was vicious. She lashed out at Janessa with no provocation, raising eyebrows and speculation among the rest of the staff. On Monday she seemed like a different person.

"Janessa, I'm glad you're working here today. You know exactly what to do in this department. Those rookie nurse's the administration sends down here should go back and take a Nursing 101 class. They simply don't have a clue and I don't have time to train people."

"Thank you, Terry. It's good to work with you too." Janessa spoke slowly and cautiously. "I know what you mean about having to train nurses in the middle of a crisis. There are always bad results when that happens."

Terry beamed at her. "Yes, that's so true. By the way, I'm really sorry about the way I acted the other day when I came in. I was stressed and

I took it out on you. Things are better now. I was confused, but I've figured things out and know what I have to do going forward."

Janessa smiled back. She thought the other nurse looked and sounded calmer than she had previously, but she couldn't help but wonder what had changed for her. "I'm glad things are working out for you. Sometimes when we're under pressure we might do something we'll regret later." Janessa could have kicked herself for saying that. She didn't want to antagonize Terry all over again by implying that she'd done something wrong. However, the other nurse seemed unfazed by what Janessa had said.

"You're so right, but things will be much better from now on. I know exactly what I have to do to maintain my equilibrium."

What an odd thing to say. After a quick smile at Terry, she moved into room two so that she could care for a young man with a possible fractured ankle. Within minutes Janessa forgot about Terry and her strange comments as she lost herself in caring for her young patient.

After work on Thursday, Janessa waited on her front step for Margarite to arrive. The women decided to walk to the fitness center to the self-defense class. After a while, Margarite arrived, parked her car in Janessa's driveway, and looked her friend up and down.

"You don't look any the worse for your encounter with the volatile Ms. Meyers. I take it she behaved this time while you were in the department?"

"Believe it or not Terry was very friendly and outgoing. Maybe we've been wrong about her all along. Maybe she was just having a bad day and took it out on the first person she ran into."

"Huh. Don't count on it. She'll be back to her old self the next time you see her. I think she might have some kind of undiagnosed mental disorder. You need to be careful around her. I don't trust her. She'll turn on you in a heartbeat."

Janessa laughed and fell in step with her friend. "You might be right, but I think I'll give her the benefit of the doubt. I don't have to work in her department for a while, so she doesn't have to see me unless the department becomes short-staffed again. Occasionally I will be filling in while Brenda is still out on maternity leave, but there are other nurses filling in, as well."

"I'm glad you're not there all the time. I need you with me so that I don't talk myself out of this ancestry thing. I'm scared about what I'll find."

"You'll be fine. I'll be with you every step of the way. Now let's go kick the self-defense instructor's butt."

They walked into the classroom together. Lance Halen and Pete Cranston were already in the room checking off the participants' names. Janessa returned Lance's smile and then took her seat without looking at Pete Cranston. After everyone checked in and sat down, the instructors stood in front of the classroom. Lance was the first to speak.

"Tonight, ladies and gentlemen we're going to teach you basic defense moves. The first one is about freeing yourself from someone who has a grip on your wrist. It doesn't matter whether it's right or left. You should be able to get away from them with the simple technique we're about to show you."

Margarite looked at Janessa. "Pay attention. You never know."

Chapter Twenty-Nine

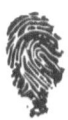

When the women returned to Janessa's house after class, they found the front door partially open. "What the?" She felt Margarite grabbing her arm to keep her from entering the house. "Margarite! Let go. Brutus, oh my God, Brutus! I have to find him! He's in there. He might be hurt!"

"Janessa, wait! Whoever broke in might still be there. We need to call the police!"

"You call them. I need to find Brutus." Janessa lightly tapped the door, which swung open. The destruction of her living room was sickening. She flicked on the light switch and called for her dog.

"Brutus, Brutus. Where are you, boy? Brutus, come to Mama." She heard a soft whine coming from the bathroom. When she opened the door, the little dog jumped into her arms. "Brutus. Thank God you're okay." The little dog rained doggie kisses on her face. The shower curtain dangled from two remaining hooks and the medicine cabinet mirror cracked beyond repair hung precariously. Janessa slowly backed out of the bathroom and turned to go into the living room, the dog in her arms. "Oh my God, who would do this?" Her gaze traveled around the room. Pictures were torn off the wall, and anything on a flat surface now lay smashed on the floor. The cushions on the couch and chair lay in tatters on the floor. Janessa ran out of the front door to wait for the police. She hadn't heard anyone inside, but the vandal could still be there, hiding. She didn't bother checking further in the house, just in case. As long as she had Brutus and he was okay, nothing else mattered.

Minutes later Detective Jim Green and a uniformed officer screeched to a halt in Janessa's driveway. After glancing at the two women huddled together at the edge of the small lawn, they crept into the house, guns drawn. The house was small, so it took only a short amount of time to search. Whoever had trashed the place was long gone.

"You're all clear Ms. Williams. I hope you have another place to stay tonight. It's not safe here and it looks like the person or persons wrecked everything in the house. Our forensics team will want to go over everything, so they'll be here for a while. Looks like they broke out the window on the back door to gain entry. Can you think of anyone who would want to harm you or destroy your property?"

Janessa shook her head no and clutched her dog to her chest. "I can't think of anyone who would do this. I mean... why would someone want to destroy everything I've worked for?"

"I can't answer that, Ma'am. I found this on the table in the kitchen. Do you know who would leave this for you and what it might mean?" He held up a scrap of paper, which was in a small bag. She and Margarite leaned close to read the message. *"Nosy people get what they deserve. Stop what you're doing or next time it won't just be your house."*

She shuddered and heard Margarite emit a gasp. "I...I have no idea who would do this to me. I don't understand that message. Nosy? I don't know I...Oh my God. This might have something to do with Lara's murder. Lara Scutterby was my patient when, she was killed."

"I heard about the Scutterby case." The detective folded his arms across his chest. He stared at her without saying anything. She knew that look. He thought she'd done this to her own house. She reached out a hand to him. She tried to hide the trembling. "I don't know what else to say. A few weeks ago, a car almost hit me when I was walking my dog. I don't know if it was related or not. I have been asking questions about Lara's death. Someone wants me to take the blame for the murder, but I won't let that happen. Obviously, I'm getting too close to the truth."

"The truth? What is the truth?"

"I haven't killed anyone and I'm doing all I can to prove it. Instead of focusing on me, the police need to find the real killer."

"I see. Well, I'll give this to Detectives Halen and Cranston. They can sort it out with you later. I've done all I can for now. Come into the station tomorrow and make out a report." He pulled a card from his pocket. "Here's the number of a cleaning service. Your homeowner's insurance might cover the cost of replacing whatever's destroyed."

"Can I go inside?"

"It's not safe, and the crime scene techs need to finish their job. When they're done you can go inside to get essentials, but you're not going to like what you see. Don't touch anything until our team finishes. As I said, you can't stay here. If you have any more trouble tonight don't hesitate to call. In the meantime, we'll see you at the station tomorrow." He looked back at the house. "I don't know how long the team will be in there. We'll make sure we have someone board up the window."

Janessa turned to Margarite when she felt a touch on her arm. She didn't realize tears were streaming down her face until her friend handed her a tissue. "Come on Nessa. Let's go to my place. You can crash there as long as you need."

"Clothes. I have no clean clothes and I'm supposed to work tomorrow."

"We'll take care of that later. I'll call the hospital for you. There's no way you can go in tomorrow and concentrate on the job."

The next day, Janessa walked into her kitchen. Every condiment, flour, and sugar on the floor crunched under her shoes as she walked across the room. The refrigerator door swung open. Everything in it had been pulled out and smashed on the tile.

Before Janessa could finish looking over the kitchen, she slid to the floor sobbing. She was shocked at the wanton destruction of her property by a person who intended to destroy her and her little house. She called the cleaning company as well as her insurance company, but the feeling of violation persisted. When she'd made her statement at the police station, she knew they didn't hold out much hope of finding the person or persons who'd trashed her house. The forensics team hadn't found any fingerprints or other evidence. They promised to call her if they came up with anything. Janessa told the police that they should check with her neighbor, Gladys Ketcham who saw everything. Chances are she saw someone entering the house or leaving it.

Janessa forced herself to get off the floor and start cleaning up the mess. She'd just grabbed the broom when her cell phone rang.

"Janessa, you'll never guess."

"What is it, Margarite? I'm not in the mood for guessing games right now. I'm waiting for the cleaning company to come and clean up this mess. Then I have a contractor coming to assess the damage to the rest of the house."

Her friend sounded like she'd been running and was out of breath. Janessa realized Margarite could barely contain her excitement.

"Charlie called. We were right, Cranston is related to Scutterby. I know your place is still a mess. Come back to my place and I'll tell you all about it. There's more than just the fact that Cranston is Scutterby's nephew."

"Nephew? That's right. You told me that before. I'll be right over."

Chapter Thirty

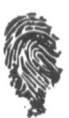

Janessa ran into Margarite's apartment. She was out of breath from jogging over instead of driving. Straining to catch her breath, she gasped as she tried to suck air into her burning lungs. *So much for getting in shape with self-defense class.* When she could talk, Janessa flopped down onto Margarite's couch and stared at her friend. "Start from the beginning. I thought I heard you say that Cranston is Leo Scutterby's nephew. How can that be? I thought Scutterby was an only child."

Margarite smirked. "Huh. A lot you know. Leo's uncle remarried when Leo was a young man. His step aunt had a young son. The two hit it off and became close. Leo and his nephew Pete are still close. Therefore, when Uncle Leo called Pete with the news about Lara, he came running, determined to catch the person who killed his cousin."

"In other words, he was and is determined to catch me and make an example of me although I didn't kill her."

"Exactly. Uncle Leo pointed the finger at you and nephew Pete jumped on the accuse Nurse Janessa bandwagon."

Janessa chewed her lower lip. "This is so unfair. I tried to take care of her, not kill her. If I could just talk to Leo and make him see reason."

"That's never going to happen. We must figure out something else."

"Well, we need to figure it out fast. I have a feeling that things are going to come crashing to a halt sooner rather than later. And I'm going to be on the receiving end of whatever bad thing happens. Whoever this person is, they're targeting me in a big way."

Janessa heard Margarite sigh. "I'm afraid you're right. Hey, I believe I can talk to Cranston. I think he likes me. As in, he really likes me. If I can sidle up to him a little more, I might get information from him as well as drop subtle hints that you're not a murderer."

Laughing, Janessa gestured to Margarites kitchen. "Got any cold water? I'm not in the mood for coffee, tea, or a soft drink. Besides, they take too much time to drink, and I need to get back to the hellhole."

Margarite went into her kitchen and opened the fridge. She grabbed a bottle of water for both of them. "Have you heard anything from Detective Hunky?"

"Lance?"

"Who else fits that description? Has he been in touch since someone destroyed your place? It's obvious someone doesn't like you poking around asking questions."

"Haven't heard a word from him."

Margarite flopped onto her couch. "Wow, I thought he would tear up the streets trying to get to you. I'm sure he's heard about it by now. I wonder what he's thinking."

Janessa headed for the door. "Obviously, he's not thinking about me. I haven't seen or heard anything from him. How about you? Anything from Cranston?"

"No and that's so odd. I' wonder if the good 'ole' boys on the scene even bothered to make a report. The one talking to you was a nasty piece of work."

"He sure was, as soon as he found out I was a person of interest in Lara's murder. Word travels fast through the police department. They had to make a report though. Forensics was there gathering evidence, but Lance and Cranston either don't know or are ignoring us. I guess we're not that important to them."

Margarite stood and walked to the door where Janessa was standing, ready to leave. "My guess is that they either haven't heard or they're on a case that's got them tied up twenty-four seven. I doubt they would ignore it when your life might be in danger."

Janessa remembered the note the other detective had found the night of the break-in. "Probably. Okay, so let's give some thought to your cozying up to Cranston. We have our next-to-the-last self-defense class on Thursday so you'd better cozy quickly. That's less than a week away. If I were you, I'd have my questions planned ahead of time."

Margarite stood in the doorway as Janessa walked out and headed toward the stairs leading to the courtyard entrance. "They say that I'm the fastest cozier this side of the Clam River."

Janessa stopped walking and turned back to her friend. "You're kidding, right?"

"What?"

"That's not a real place, is it? The Clam River? Is that really a thing?"

"I beg your pardon, it really is. It's a small river that runs next to a bar in lower Connecticut near my folk's place."

Janessa resumed her walk to the stairs. "Wow. Who would have thought it was real, with a name like that. Well, I'll be. See you tomorrow. We're in the Unit together. Seems like it's been a long time, but I know it hasn't been. So much has happened in the last few days."

"When do you work with the crazy woman again?"

"Terry?" At Margarite's nod, Janessa continued. "I have to check the schedule, but I think I'm working in the emergency Department next Tuesday and Wednesday, 7 A to 7 P."

"You need to be careful with that one. She's odd, and I don't trust her. She knows more about Lara's death than what she's saying."

"Um," Janessa agreed. "That and her out of control temper tantrums because I'm working there. I don't mind working with someone who's a flake, but she's over the limit weird."

Margarite laughed. "I'll say. She's three tomatoes short of a salad."

Janessa laughed, gave a backward wave, and opened the door to the stairway. "Haven't heard that one before. I'll see you tomorrow. Early!"

Margarite's "See you tomorrow," was barely audible as the door closed behind Janessa.

The air was chilly, although it was still afternoon. She dreaded facing her little house again with the mountain of cleaning she had to do. Even with the cleaning service coming to help, the amount was overwhelming. As Janessa neared her house, she saw someone waiting in front of her door. She was still too far away to see who it was. Her steps slowed. She had to admit to herself that she was frightened after seeing what someone had done to her house and the warning they'd left. Janessa was sure she didn't know enough self-defense to protect herself adequately. She hoped it was just a friendly neighbor checking on her to see if she was okay.

As she got closer, she could see that the person on her front step was a man. *Lance.* It was as if she and Margarite had conjured him up by talking about him. He was the last person she expected to see on her doorstep.

"Lance, what are you doing here? I wasn't expecting to see you."

He didn't say a word as he folded her into his arms and held her tight. "I'm here now. I wish I could have come sooner, but Pete Cranston and I have been on a stakeout for the past few nights. I came as soon as we had that case under control. I'm here now, sweetheart."

Janessa's shock was fading, but she held tight to him. She was exactly where she wanted to be, in Lance Halen's arms.

Chapter Thirty-One

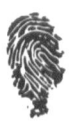

Friday at work went by quickly. She and Margarite had been busy during their shift. Janessa was able to get into her house and get clothes for work. Her house still needed repairs and she couldn't move back in yet. Saturday and Sunday flew by. Janessa was still reveling in the fact that as soon as they caught Lara's killer, she and Lance could be together. He'd stayed and helped her clean her house. The cleaning crew was due to come and finish the major portion, but Janessa was impatient. She wanted to be comfortable in her home again. That couldn't happen until the techs collected all the evidence of the vandalism. The spare bedroom was still off limits. It would take a while, but she was determined to get her little house back the way it had been before the destruction.

On Tuesday and Wednesday, Janessa worked in the Emergency department without any further incidents. In fact, Terry had been quite pleasant. She was at Janessa's side to help and even offered sound advice with the most critical patients. "You're a good nurse, Terry. Thank you for all your help." Janessa said on her last day in the ER.

"No, thank *you*. Getting slammed like we did was no picnic. Having you here was a God send. When I get someone who doesn't know the department, it makes it harder to get anything done including treating patients."

When Janessa left the Emergency Department, she was troubled. Terry had seemed so normal. The belligerence she'd displayed previously was no longer there. *I can't wait to tell Margarite about the last two days. She's not going to believe Terry's attitude.* Janessa finished her shift, clocked out, and drove the short distance to her house. A short time later she entered her front door. The house was almost back to normal. New furniture and a paint job went a long way to restore the house and Janessa's equilibrium. She's even had the kitchen tiles replaced because the condiments stained the grout between the tiles. Brutus wrapped his little body around her legs until she picked him up. She's left him at doggy daycare, so they hadn't seen much of each other. They exchanged several doggy and human kisses before she put him on the floor.

Her cell phone rang as she hung her jacket on the rack by the door. "Hi, Margarite. I was just about to call you. I love caller ID. I don't have to talk to anyone I don't like."

"Glad to hear you like me. How were your two days with Terry the Terrible?"

"Terrific."

"What? "Margarite asked. "Don't tell me you had a good time working with her. This is Terry we're talking about? The one who wanted to slap the brown color off your face?"

Janessa laughed. "Yes. The same Terry. I guess she's back on whatever meds she was taking. She was very cordial and helpful on both days when I was there. She even thanked me for coming down to the department to help."

"You're kidding. What happened to her? She's been a witch every time you worked there and suddenly; she's treating you like you're her good buddy. Why? Something's not right."

Janessa sighed and walked into the kitchen and opened the back door so that Brutus could go out into the fenced area. "It's only eight o'clock. Why don't you come over for supper? We can order a pizza and talk. We need to re-plan our strategy and discuss this change that's come over Terry. I don't know if it's going to last and it's very confusing."

"I'll be there in ten minutes. Go ahead and order the pizza. That way we won't have to wait too long before it's delivered. I'm starved."

"Me too. I want veggies on my half. Pepperoni on yours?"

"You bet. See you shortly."

A short time later, Margarite arrived, and not long after that the pizza and soda arrived. Janessa fed Brutus, admonished him about begging, and then set the table for her and Margarite. Between bites of pizza and sips of soda, the two women discussed Lara's murder and Terry's overnight personality change. Margarite swallowed her last bit of food and said, "I'm not buying Terry's sweet act. Are you? I mean she's been beyond mean and nasty, and now suddenly, she's nice and helpful. Why? Is she the one who trashed your house and now she feels that she's scared you off your investigation of Lara's death?"

"I agree. Trashing my house was the second attack on me. I didn't connect the two at first, but now I'm beginning to wonder."

Margarite looked puzzled. "Second attack?"

"Yes. Remember I told you about the car that ran me and Brutus off the road when we went for our walk one night?" At Margarite's nod, she continued. "I think that was the first time whoever it was tried to scare me."

"Do you think it was Terry? I know you couldn't see the driver and we don't know what kind of car she drives, but..." Margarite asked before taking a hefty drink of soda from her glass.

Janessa was quiet then she sighed and looked at her friend. "I just don't know. It's like my house. Someone trashed it but why? The only motive I can think of is that someone doesn't want me looking into Lara's murder. Perhaps it's the murderer."

"Well, there are a few people we can automatically rule out." Margarite set her glass on the table and continued. "Leo for one. I don't think he'd have the stamina to destroy your house. Plus, he was in the hospital when you were nearly run over by that car. We can eliminate Lance, of course. He's crazy about you." Janessa felt her face get hot, but she let her friend continue. "I think we can also eliminate Pete Cranston. He seems to be a by-the-book cop. He might want to put you in jail, but I can't see him terrorizing you like this. Also, I don't think he had moved here when you had the car incident."

Janessa shook her head, got up to put the dishes in the sink, and sat back down at the table. "So, we're back at square one. We have no suspect for either incident and no suspect for Lara's murder."

"Oh yes, we do."

Janessa studied her friend, who wore a serious expression on her face, which was unusual for Margarite. She was usually the one who did the laughing and joking. Janessa was the more serious one of the two.

"Terry."

"I'm still not sure. She is odd, I admit that. But murder? Why? What does she have to gain by murdering a patient, who by all accounts she barely knew."

"It fits and she had access to Lara. She also could have been driving, spotted you, and decided to kill two birds with one stone, so to speak. And your address is known to almost anyone who cares to find you. I think she's guilty."

Janessa stood up and paced the small area. "Maybe she is, but..." She looked at her friend. "I keep coming back to one question. Why?"

Chapter Thirty-Two

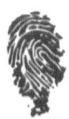

On Thursday Janessa unexpectedly had to work in the Emergency department. Someone had called out sick, so the nursing supervisor sent Janessa to fill in.

"I don't understand why they keep making you work down there. Don't we have any other cross-trained nurses?" Margarite asked unsympathetically.

"Potts says I'm the only one on who's familiar with the emergency department's routines. Besides, I don't mind. I have an idea that I haven't investigated before. I'm hoping I'll get a chance to snoop."

Margarite rolled her eyes. "Be careful! Especially if you're working with crazy Terry. Are you? Working with her?"

Janessa didn't answer. She gathered her things and headed for the elevator. She felt guilty that she had to desert Margarite in the critical care unit, although it was quiet with only one non-critical patient.

"You are, aren't you? You're working with that lunatic. Be careful. I don't want to have to plan your funeral."

Janessa turned, smiled, and waved to her friend. The elevator door closed, and she rode to the lower level. She exited the elevator and walked down the corridor to the emergency department. She was hoping to get access to the AMD, Automated Drug Dispenser logs for the night Lara died. She suspected that someone had overridden the system, pulled up a fatal dose of Sodium Chloride, and then administered it to Lara Scutterby through her IV. The drug was available on the crash cart, but according to the medical examiner, Lara's dose was extremely high. There was only one way to get that much of the drug. The woman didn't have a chance. The good thing, if there was anything good, was that Lara would have felt almost nothing before she died.

The emergency department was busy when Janessa walked in. By the time she'd gotten to the department, Huddle was over. She got a brief report from the director and then went into cubicle three to tend to a severe leg laceration. A sixteen-year-old male fell off a bike and onto a pile of glass. The left leg was flayed open exposing all the layers down to the bone. She began cleaning the wound after she called the on-duty surgeon. She had just finished the final wound cleanse when Scott Wilkins strode into the cubicle.

"Let's see what we have here." He looked at the patient notes Janessa had made on the computer. "Jeremy, you really did a number on yourself, didn't you?" Dr. Wilkins said. "We're going to wash this out one more time, then we'll numb it a little bit so that I can sew you back up. What were you doing to cut yourself like that?"

Jeremy looked at the doctor then looked away, his face reddening. "I was riding my bike. I hit a rock and went over the handlebars into a pile of glass. When I got up, my leg was spitting blood everywhere. Will I have a scar?"

"I'm afraid so," said the doctor. Your cut goes through all the skin layers to the bone. We'll give you some antibiotics when we're done so that you don't get an infection."

Janessa had everything assembled for the doctor to stitch Jeremy's leg. She knew it would take a while. The cut was deep and long. "Do your parents know where you are, Jeremy?"

He looked at Janessa and grinned. "Yeah, I called them before the ambulance picked me up. My mom is in full panic mode, but she's on her way here. My dad is still at work, but I'm sure by now my mom has called him so he might show up here too." At that moment there was a commotion as Terry pulled the curtain open in the cubicle. A short, thin woman Janessa assumed was Jeremy's mother pushed her way in.

"Jeremy! Are you okay? You hung up so fast I couldn't make head or tail...Oh my God! What happened? How did this happen?"

Jeremy's mother was at the head of the gurney, her hand on Jeremy's shoulder. Janessa could see that her hand was shaking. The doctor glanced at the papers Janessa had handed him minutes earlier. "Mrs. Paxton, I'm going to flush the wound again to make sure there are no glass particles in there. I don't think the wound warrants a trip to the operating room. Once I'm sure the wound is clear, I'll stitch him up, give him a prescription for antibiotics, and he'll be fine. Is that all right with you?" At her nod yes, he continued. "No bike riding for a while though."

Jeremy's mother offered a faint smile. "No way. This young man will be housebound for a while, and we will park that bike."

"It needs to be fixed anyway," Jeremy mumbled, while his mother patted his arm.

The doctor numbed Jeremy's leg with an injection. After getting seventy-six stitches and a dose of antibiotics, Jeremy was ready for discharge. "The inner stitches will dissolve on their own, Mrs. Paxton. Take him to your regular doctor in a couple of weeks to get it checked and have the rest of the stitches removed. Watch for any redness or discolored fluid oozing from the wound. Until the stitches come out, cover it with plastic when he showers. He shouldn't get it wet for at least a week. Jeremy, the stitches will start itching in the next few days as they heal, but *absolutely no scratching*. Are you clear about what I've said?"

At the boy's nod, his mother placed her hand on his cheek. "Nothing to worry about Doctor. I'll make sure he does everything you've asked him to do. My husband is probably here now, so if you're done with Jeremy, we'll be on our way."

Dr Wilkins handed her a prescription. "This is for antibiotics. Make sure he takes them as directed and that he finishes the bottle."

Janessa cleaned up after Jeremy's visit, then decided she had time to make a quick visit to her friend Paulie who worked in the pharmacy. She called out to Terry and told her she'd be right back, that she had a quick errand to run.

Paulie was behind the half door of the pharmacy, filling an order for an employee who stood nearby. "Hey, Nessa, what's up?"

Janessa smiled at the tall, thin young pharmacist. He'd been on staff for nearly a year, and they'd become firm friends within the first two weeks. She hesitated before asking him what she wanted him to do, but she couldn't think of any other way to go about it. She waited until the employee left the area. "Paulie, I want to ask you to do something for me. Feel free to say no because it's a little unethical. If anyone finds out, you could be in trouble. So, if you don't feel comfortable doing it, speak up and refuse. I won't be angry with you, I'll understand. I promise."

"Spit it out before someone comes and overhears us. If I'm going to lose my job, I don't want the entire hospital to know. What is it?"

Janessa looked up and down the hallway. No one was there. "You have access to the AMD, right? You can review the logs of all the meds dispensed?"

Paulie stared at Janessa "You know I do. What do you need?"

"This goes back a while." She gave him the date of Lara's admission. I need to know if there was an override of Sodium Chloride that night. A large dose"

He whistled. "Sodium Chloride? Normally no one pays attention to something like that, but a large dose? That's unusual."

"A dose big enough to kill."

"Oh brother, Janessa, what are you getting yourself into?"

"I told you that you could refuse to do this. I don't want you to get into trouble. Here's my cell phone number. Call me later today when our shifts are over. I don't want to take a chance on anyone overhearing us."

"Okay, you've got it."

"Thanks, Paulie. I owe you one." She turned to go back to the emergency room.

"Oh and 'Nessa?"

Janessa turned to look at him. "Don't be such a stranger. I hardly see you anymore." He grinned and she turned away with a quick wave.

She walked into the Emergency Department where things were still quiet. Terry flounced into the nurse's station and threw herself into the next chair. She stared intently at Janessa. "Okay, so where did you have to go in such a rush?"

Janessa was trying to figure out what she could say when Terry continued. "What was so important at the pharmacy?"

Chapter Thirty-Three

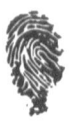

J anessa stammered and sputtered her way through the encounter with Terry. After mumbling something about not seeing her friend for a long time, she escaped. That was too close for comfort. She still wasn't sure about Terry's involvement in Lara's death, but she had her suspicions. The woman was always one step behind Janessa when she was investigating. It was uncomfortable. She still wasn't sure if Terry was the killer or not.

Either way, she didn't want to be alone with her. As soon as her shift finished, Janessa made her way to the parking lot and hopped into her Mini Cooper. As she pulled out onto the street, she noticed a car following close behind her. She couldn't be sure if it was the same car that ran her and Brutus off the road a few weeks ago. She'd only seen the bright headlights and the barest glimpse of the tinted windows.

Janessa took a series of sharp turns hoping she could lose the car behind her, but it didn't work. The car stayed on her bumper. The drive to her small house was short, but she drove past it. No way would she be trapped in her house with a killer if that's who was following her. She had another destination in mind. After barely putting on her turn signal, she abruptly pulled into the parking lot at the police station. She spotted an open parking space close to the door of the building. Janessa glanced in her rearview mirror as the other car sped past.

She had to decide whether to go in and report the incident or drive out of the parking lot and head to the doggy daycare to pick up Brutus then go home, taking a chance that whoever was driving that car wasn't waiting for her down the road. To heck with that. She opened her car door and got out. She'd rather make a fool of herself in the police station than risk her life and not report it.

When Janessa marched into the police station, she heaved a sigh of relief when she spotted Lance, her would-be boyfriend. He smiled and waved her over to the desk then looked at her face and hurried around to her side of the desk.

"Janessa, what's wrong? You look like you've seen a ghost. You're trembling too."

Suddenly everything that had happened in the last few minutes caught up with her. She began to shake. Tears weren't far away. She could feel the sting in her eyes.

"I ... someone was following me." The tears threatened to fall with each word she uttered.

"Take your time, Babe. You're safe now." Lance put his arm around her and drew her close. At that moment Detective Pete Cranston walked into the front of the police station from the back room. He cleared his throat.

"What's going on here? Do I have to remind you Detective that this is a police station and not a..."

"Stow it, Pete. Janessa's upset. Someone tailed her from work. Now be quiet and let me get the whole story."

Pete was quiet while Lance gently walked Janessa over to a chair and made her sit down. He sat beside her, and Pete Cranston hovered nearby. "Take your time and tell me what happened."

Janessa hiccupped, fumbled for a tissue in her pocket, and blew her nose. "I just left work. As soon as I drove out of the hospital parking lot and turned onto Elm Street, I noticed a car behind me. It was too close. I turned onto a couple of different roads to see if I could escape, but the car stayed on my bumper. I can't be sure if it was the same car that knocked Brutus and me into a ditch one night when we were out walking. When I drove into the parking lot here, the car sped away. I couldn't get a look at the driver. I didn't want to go home without telling the police in case anything else happened. I don't want a repeat of what happened to my house the other night, especially with me inside."

Detective Cranston stared at her. "Tell me about being thrown into a ditch."

Janessa couldn't help but smile at his phraseology.

"My dog Brutus and I were out for a walk one night not too long ago. We were nearing my house when a car suddenly came behind us from out of nowhere. It was traveling fast and was close to us. I only had time to scoop Brutus into my arms and dive into the ditch. That's the only thing that saved us. The car had dark windows and was speeding so I couldn't see who was driving it or get a license plate number. I'm fairly sure it was the same car today. Dark windows and no front plate."

"Did you see any identifying marks that you can remember?" Lance asked, still sitting next to her. He had his arm across the back of the chair.

"Not really. Everything happened too fast. I just wanted to get here and get away from whoever was driving that car. I don't know if this is related to the vandalism at my house or not. It might be the same person or someone different."

Lance stood and walked to the desk. He picked up a notepad and walked back over to Janessa. "Write down everything you can remember. Even the smallest detail could be helpful. Someone has it in for you and we'd like to try and figure out why."

Detective Cranston moved closer. "Has anything out of the ordinary happened lately? Other than the vandalism at your house, I mean. Anything different at work?"

Janessa felt her face heat. She wasn't sure if she should tell them about what she'd asked her friend Paulie in the pharmacy to do for her. She didn't want to get him into any trouble or worse, risk him losing his job. She hesitated, wondering how to answer without implicating him. "I have been checking to see who overrode the Automated Med

Dispenser on the night that Lara died. Someone ordered a large dose of Sodium Chloride that night. No patients were on that medication. It's a specialty drug. There's a way to look at the records for that night and see who signed for it. That person is possibly the killer. It's the only way I know to catch them, then the police can take over."

Detective Cranston and Lance exploded at the same time; however, Detective Cranston's voice was loudest. "And you didn't think to tell us about this until now that your life is in danger? No wonder someone's trying to kill you."

Chapter Thirty-Four

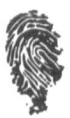

Janessa cringed, not used to having voices raised against her. "I know, I know. I just thought..."

"That's just it, you didn't think." Pete Cranston's face was beet red. His rage was palpable.

Why is he so angry? It's a little out of proportion. She shifted in her seat and stole a glance at Lance. His features were rigid, and it was hard to tell what he was thinking. "I didn't do anything wrong if you remember. I just wanted to report what happened in case you find my dead body and have no idea what happened to me."

"I could give you a couple of good reasons," Pete mumbled under his breath.

A sharp look from Lance stopped Pete. He turned away and walked over to the desk and sat down. He didn't say another word, just watched Janessa and Lance. He made her uncomfortable, so she turned away from his unrelenting stare.

"Relax, Janessa," Lance said. "We understand. Let's see if we can figure out who has you in their sights and why. Have you had any disagreements with anyone lately?"

"Not really. I mean there's a nurse at Ashton Community who is angry that I've been asking questions about Lara Scutterby's death." She risked a glance at Pete Cranston and saw his frown. She figured he still considered her guilty of the woman's death. Other than that, it's been business as usual."

"Do you understand that you're not the police? What did you think you were doing investigating a murder on your own?" Pete

Cranston sputtered. His face was bright red with anger. "You need to stay out of this and let us do our job."

"Look. I know you're angry with me, Detective Cranston, but my life and reputation are on the line. I'm a suspect in the murder of a woman I never met until the night someone killed her. I couldn't sit back and do nothing when the police focused solely on me because of Leo Scutterby's influence. He's done nothing but bad mouth and accuse me when I had nothing to do with Lara's death. I tried my best and did my job trying to save her." Janessa was nearly shouting. Tears stung her eyes. She'd forced herself to unclench her fists.

She saw Lance and Pete exchange a look before eyeing Janessa. "We know, Janessa. We are actively investigating Lara's case. You're not the only one we've focused on. I know it feels that way, but we are trying to figure out who killed Lara Scutterby too and why."

Janessa sniffed. She wasn't normally an emotional wreck, but fear and frustration were taking their toll on her. "I just feel like I'm under the spotlight for her death. I work hard to help my patients get well. I would never intentionally hurt anyone. Especially someone I didn't even know. Her father needs to know that. I have no idea if he's behind the person who keeps targeting me or not, but it's frightening to have someone follow me, trash my house, and almost run over me and my dog."

Lance patted her shoulder. "I want you to go home, lock your doors, and let us manage this. We can't focus on who is doing what to whom if we are busy trying to be bodyguards working to keep you safe. Can you do that? Can you go home and stay there until you need to leave for work tomorrow? Keep your eyes and ears open. We'll do extra patrols by your house."

"But I ... that is, tonight is..."

"Ms. Williams is trying to tell you that tonight is Thursday. Self-defense class is tonight." Pete looked at Janessa and nodded.

"Yes. I need to be able to go. Margarite will expect to attend the class. We travel together so I won't be alone. The class is almost at an end and it's important to us that we finish it."

Pete and Lance exchanged another look that Janessa couldn't interpret so she gave up trying. She was determined to go to class tonight. She needed all the self-defense tactics she could learn in the event of a personal attack. The way things were happening to her, there was a likelihood of that event. If the police started looking at other people, they might find the real killer and Janessa could get on with her life.

Janessa stood up to leave the police station. "I'm going home now. I'm sure Brutus is anxious to go home, and I need to pick him up at doggy daycare. I need to feed him before I get ready for tonight's class. I will be there. I've learned techniques, but I have more to learn to protect myself. Listen, you might not believe me, but I know there's a threat out there and I'm a target. I'm guessing that whoever is doing these things to me is probably Lara's killer."

Pete Cranston walked around behind the desk and sat down. After making a note he looked up. "Okay, Ms. Williams. Go home and do what you need to do. We'll see you tonight."

"Thank you. I will see you both later. I'll call Margarite and have her come to my house. That way we can leave for the class together."

"Good idea." Lance walked her to the door. His warm hand resting on the small of her back made Janessa conscious of his touch. If she hadn't been so upset by the events, she would have been over the moon with his attention. "Stay aware of your surroundings. Be prepared for anything especially when you're driving."

"I will. Thank you for listening to me. I'll see you tonight." Janessa left the police station and started the drive home. She took a deep breath. *Maybe I'll have help with this now.* She picked up Brutus from daycare, drove home, and pulled into her driveway.

THE DETECTIVES STARED after the retreating woman. Lance looked over at Pete. "What do you think, Pete? Any ideas?"

"We have a real dilemma on our hands. A couple of weeks ago I would have bet money on Janessa Williams being guilty in my cousin's death. Now? She bears watching for a different reason. Someone is trying to kill the only witness we have in Lara's death."

Chapter Thirty-Five

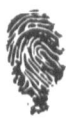

J anessa called Margarite as soon as she got home from the police station. She kept looking in her rearview mirror, but there were no further incidents of any cars following her. She fed Brutus and let him out into the gated backyard. "Sorry, little guy. No walk for us tonight. Orders from our esteemed police detectives." The little dog cocked his head at her then lunged for the back door. *I guess no walk is okay with you tonight.* She opened the door for the little dog to go out.

After Brutus finished his business and came back inside, he nosed his food dish toward Janessa. She fed him his kibble, refreshed his water, and then walked into her bedroom to change into something suitable for a self-defense class. This was their next to the last class, but she still didn't feel prepared if anything happened. She finished dressing then went back to the kitchen and made a chef's salad for her dinner. She didn't want to eat anything too heavy because of the physical activity they would be doing in the classroom. After the events of the day, she had little appetite. She picked at her small salad.

Janessa had just finished eating when her cell phone rang. Paulie Standard, her pharmacist friend in Ashton Hospital, was on the one calling. "Hey, 'Nessa, you were right. Someone did override the AMD on the night you questioned. They signed out a double dose of Sodium Chloride. Given that amount, it's doubtful you'd ever wake up."

"I knew it. So, who was it? Who signed for it?" Janessa could feel her excitement building. She was hot on the trail of a killer and now she was close to knowing who it was.

"That's the odd thing," Paulie said. "No one signed for it. There's no signature. What I mean is that there is a scribbled initial that's unreadable. I tried backtracking before and after the withdrawal and I didn't find a thing. Someone ghosted the machine. How? I don't know, but I intend to find out. You're not supposed to be able to sign out anything without a complete signature. Putting in an illegible initial is not only unacceptable, but it's also illegal."

Janessa drew in a deep breath. "Please be careful. We're up against a ruthless killer who doesn't care about anyone. This person killed a helpless patient so anyone getting in the way is probably fair game. And for God's sake if you talk to Potts or Doane, do yourself a favor and don't mention my name. It will be easier for you. I am persona non grata and Bully Bill would love to get another report on me."

"Okay. I'll keep you out of it. I collate the logs for the AMD so my spotting an irregularity like that won't raise any red flags. I'll keep you posted."

Janessa clicked off her phone. How frustrating. *We are so close.* She knew Margarite would be there shortly, so she sat down to wait for her friend. She felt a tap on her leg and looked down to see Brutus with his water bowl in his mouth, tapping at her leg. "You silly dog," she laughed. "Okay, I'll refill your water bowl. I'm sorry you ran out of water. I'm a neglectful mommy." A short rap on the door signaled the arrival of her friend.

"What's up?" Margarite asked. "I thought we were meeting at the center for the self-defense class. I'm glad I got your text early enough to come here first."

Janessa stood and grabbed her jacket from the back of the chair where she'd placed it. "Let's get going so we're not late for class. I'll tell you about it on the way there."

While walking the short distance to the self-defense class, Janessa filled Margarite in on the events of the last few hours. "I knew someone would come after you." Margarite said. "What happens now? Will you keep digging? Should I start planning to contact your family so we can plan your funeral?"

Janessa had never had Margarite chastise her. Her friend was angry, and she couldn't blame her. She was probably as frightened as Janessa. "What's with you and funerals lately? No one needs to plan my funeral. Nothing is going to happen to me."

"You can't know that. This person is coming after you and more than likely they're Lara Scutterby's killer. You've asked too many questions and brought the wrong kind of attention to yourself." She stopped on the sidewalk. Janessa had no choice but to stop and look at her. "You'll be next, and I couldn't take that."

Janessa hugged her friend. "It will be okay. You'll see. I got a big lead on the killer a little while ago. Paulie called me and confirmed my suspicions. Someone overrode the AMD and took out a double dose of Sodium Chloride."

"Oh my God! You were right all along. So, who was it? That person is probably the killer, right? Did Paulie give you a name? "

"You're right, it was probably Lara's killer. However, somehow, this person managed to get the drugs without a complete signature. All my friend could find was a scribbled initial. He couldn't read it. He's going to keep checking, but he probably won't find anything. This person is ruthless." She glanced at her Fitbit watch. "We need to hustle. Class will start soon, and we still aren't there yet. God knows I don't need Cranston glaring at me all evening."

"He's not that bad. Once you get to know him." There was still enough daylight outside for Janessa to see Marguerite blush.

"You have a real soft spot for him, don't you?"

Her friend's blush might have deepened. "He asked me out."

Janessa searched her friend's face, but Margarite showed little of what she was feeling inside. "I hope you don't mind. I said yes."

"Mind? Why should I mind? You are a grown adult who can make your own decisions. The attraction has been there since the day you two met. I say go for it. However, if he doesn't treat you right, I'll put a couple of self-defense moves of my own on him. With you dating him, maybe someday he'll stop being suspicious of me. Hopefully before he decides to arrest me."

Both women laughed but sobered as they entered the classroom. Detective Cranston gave them a stern look for interrupting whatever he'd been talking about, but Janessa noticed that his gaze softened when he looked at Margarite. *Boy, he's got it bad.* She glanced at her friend, who seemed mesmerized by Pete's gaze. *Wow, she's got it as bad as he does.*

"Okay, ladies and gents. Tonight, Detective Halen and I are going to show you what to do if you're faced with an armed attacker." Janessa saw that he was looking right at her. "The moves we show you should at least keep you from getting killed and should hold off your attacker until you can either get away or help arrives." His gaze never wavered from Janessa's. "At the very least it might keep you from becoming a homicide statistic."

Chapter Thirty-Six

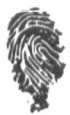

The self-defense class lasted longer than usual. When Janessa checked her watch, she saw that it had been a half hour longer than usual. However, she felt much more confident in her abilities than she had at the start of the class. She knew that didn't mean she could defend herself against all takers, but she felt she had a better chance now than before. She and Margarite walked back to Janessa's house in relative silence, each lost in her thoughts.

When the women walked into the house, Brutus who had been waiting at the door, attacked them and began dancing around Janessa's legs before darting to the kitchen door. "Hang on a minute, Margarite. Let me get this attack dog out into the backyard." She laughed as she walked into the kitchen turning on lights as she made her way through. When Brutus finished, he whined and scratched at the door. Janessa gave him a treat after she let him in and refilled his water bowl. He was content for the moment, so she went back to the living room to talk to Margarite.

"While we were in class, I got a text from Potts. She wants me to work in the emergency room tomorrow. Someone has already called out and they were short-staffed to begin with."

"Do you have to work with the 'witch?'"

"If you mean Terry, I have no idea. Maybe I'll get lucky, and she'll be the one who called out. Then, the problem is solved."

"In your dreams. You know she'll be there to torture you with her snide remarks and her sketchy ways. I said it before and I'll repeat it, I don't trust her. She's up to no good. Watch your back or maybe I should say, don't turn your back on her. I still think she's dangerous."

"You're probably right. I don't trust her either. But I have no proof that she's done anything wrong. If I could find anything, I could let our friendly neighborhood detectives know. That would get me out of Leo Scutterby's sights and ole Bully Bill wouldn't be able to accuse me of Lara's death."

"Until the next time. He's not going to let it rest until he gets to kick you out of the hospital for good. You got on his bad side when you refused to date him, so now he wants revenge."

"I know, but not only is he gross, he's married. I've never met his wife. She must be a real winner. There aren't too many women I know who want to get anywhere near him."

Margarite smiled and slowly walked to the front door. "I've met her. She's not much in the looks department, but she's an extremely nice woman. I feel sorry for her, but you know what they say about love being blind."

Janessa stood with her mouth gaping. "You're kidding. The meanest man in Ashton is married to a nice woman. Go figure. I wonder how he pulled that off. Maybe he got her drunk and proposed when she passed out or something. I can't think of anyone who would willingly tie herself to him."

"Your guess is as good as mine. Maybe he has hidden good qualities about which we don't know. She must be a saint to put up with him and his antics. That is if she knows about them. I'm sure he hides a lot from her."

"Hmm," Janessa said, walking her friend to the door. "Maybe he doesn't bully her. Could be that he's nice to her." At Margarite's skeptical look, she grinned. "Hey, you never know what goes on behind closed doors."

Margarite left after the women said their final goodnight. Janessa had to admit that she was a little nervous about her shift in the emergency room the following day. *Who knows, maybe it will be peaceful. No drama.*

The following day, Janessa reported to the emergency department. The place overflowed with patient emergencies. There was barely time to take a deep breath, let alone take a bathroom break. Many of the cases were minor ones that were resolved within minutes. Others were more complex and perplexing. They needed more advanced assessment and time to diagnose and treat them. That was the case with Mrs. Elaine Tucker. She was a slightly overweight middle-aged woman complaining of general weakness, nausea, and vomiting. Janessa, assigned to take care of the woman, began doing all the prep work before Darryl Mintz, the Physician's Assistant examined her.

"Good afternoon, Mrs. Tucker. My name is Janessa, and I will be taking care of you while you're in the emergency department. Can you tell me about your symptoms? What you're experiencing, when the problem began, that sort of thing.

Elaine Tucker moaned and reached for the basin near her hand. She retched and then vomited an amount that nearly overflowed the basin. She was unable to speak due to the vomiting, so Janessa readied the equipment she needed to start an intravenous line and do an electrocardiogram; a standard protocol for someone coming into the emergency department with Mrs. Tucker's symptoms. After she got the intravenous started, Janessa left the cubicle to empty the basin of vomit. The basins had measurement lines on them, so she'd be able to give an amount to Darryl when he came in. He was sure to ask, and Janessa was prepared.

When she returned from the bathroom, the woman seemed slightly better. The color of her face was near normal, and she wasn't sweating as much. Janessa hooked up the EKG machine and prepared to run a strip showing what Elaine's heart was doing in case she was having a heart attack. Janessa put all the leads on Elaine. She checked that the wires were okay and that everything worked properly. She pressed buttons and eventually a strip of paper with the cardiac reading came out of the machine. *I'm not a doctor, but this EKG looks normal to me. However, sometimes it takes a while for anything to show up on the monitor. Time will tell.*

Janessa finished taking the rest of Elaine's vital signs and was satisfied that everything looked like it was within normal range. Maybe the patient had a virus, but it was best to rule out everything. "I'm sorry I can't give you anything for the vomiting; I have to wait until Darryl Mintz, the Physician's Assistant examines you. I'm sure he'll order something for you that will ease your discomfort."

"It's a little better, Nurse. I've been like this off and on since yesterday afternoon. First, the pain starts in my abdomen then the vomiting begins. I haven't been able to go to work or keep anything down. I thought I'd be better by today, but it's still there."

Janessa smiled at Elaine and patted her hand. "You try to rest for now. I'm sure the PA will be in shortly. He was with another patient down the hall. But I think he'll be in to see you soon. I'll be back in a couple of minutes. In the meantime, if you need anything, push this button to signal me or any other nurse who's in the vicinity. Janessa left the cubical and sat down at the nurse's station to enter the information she'd gathered on Elaine Tucker into the computer. She took advantage of the quiet moment to go to the lady's room.

Trying to be as quick as possible, Janessa used the bathroom, washed her hands, and headed back to Elaine Tucker's cubicle to check on her. She was mindful of what happened to Lara Scutterby the minute she walked out of the room. The last thing she needed was a repeat with Elaine Tucker. She had a gut feeling that she needed to stay close to the woman.

As soon as she walked in, Janessa knew something was off. It was odd that the cubicle curtain was around the area. Certain that wasn't how she left it; she pulled the curtain back so she could see her patient. "Are you feeling... Terry, what are you doing here? And why do you have that in your hand near my patient? Drop that and get the hell away from her. Now!"

Terry Meyers stood at Elaine Tucker's bedside with a large, full syringe in her hand, poised to inject it into the patient's intravenous tube.

Chapter Thirty-Seven

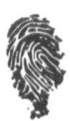

At first, Terry didn't move. She shifted back into position over Elaine Tucker's arm, the needle poised in her hand. Janessa edged closer, trying to get close enough to prevent Terry's attack on the patient. No one would die tonight if she could help it.

"Don't do it, Terry. She's innocent. She's done nothing to you. Please step away from the bed and drop the needle. You don't want to do this. Think of the consequences you'll face if you kill another patient."

"What consequences, Ms. Perfect? She is an innocent patient, but the point is that she's *your* patient. Don't you understand that? You'll be the one facing consequences when another patient of yours is found dead."

Janessa took another step forward, but Terry spotted her movement.

"Don't come any closer," she said, her hand dangerously close to Elaine's IV line. You won't have time to react. She'll be dead before you can grab my arm. I suggest you stay where you are."

"Why?" Janessa knew she had to keep the other woman talking and distracted. Praying for a miracle, she hoped someone would come into the cubicle and help before Terry killed the woman. "You'll kill me too, like you killed Lara? You did kill her, didn't you?"

"You killed Lara, didn't you?" Terry mocked her in a sing-song voice. "I had to. Don't you see? I needed her out of the way so that my father would finally pay attention to me without the distraction of his 'legal' daughter. I did it to save our relationship."

"Your father? Leo Scutterby is your father?"

"Of course. He couldn't keep it in his pants although he had a wife and child on the way. He had a fling with my mother then went on his merry way back to his wife and daughter. He left us for them and never looked back."

Janessa stood as still as a statue. She and Margarite had been so close when they'd guessed that there was another child somewhere. "Does Leo even know that you're his daughter?"

Terry snickered. "Of course not. He was so anxious to get back to his loving wife he barely asked my mother's name let alone learn that she'd had his bastard child. Sounds cliché, doesn't it? Me, a lowly emergency department nurse that no one really likes, is the bastard child of upstanding citizen, Board President Leo Scutterby."

"Okay, I get that you must be hurt by what he did. But why didn't your mother ever contact him? I think Leo would have done something to help. He might be an arrogant SOB, but he made sure that despite their estrangement Lara had everything she needed."

"God knows, my mother tried. But he and his happy family moved, and she had no idea where he was. Her letters were returned unopened. After a while, she gave up. When I turned 18, I spent my adult years tracking him down. I wanted to make him pay for all the pain he caused us. After I graduated from nursing school, I traced him to this little hole-in-the wall hospital. Getting rid of his perfect daughter seemed like a good idea. With her out of the way he's free to take care of me, his only daughter."

Focusing on her story, Terry didn't notice Janessa fumbling in her pocket. She pushed a button on her phone, praying her fingers had found the mark. *Damn, the screen lock is on.* She usually left the phone unlocked at work in case she needed to make an emergency call.

Trying to get the phone unlocked wasted time. She hoped she'd managed to push the emergency call button on the phone, which worked even with the phone locked. She couldn't look for the button, so she pushed what she thought might be the 911 emergency help button so that someone could hear Terry's rantings and maybe send help.

"But why kill this patient? She's done nothing to you. You don't even know her."

"She's *your* patient. Two dead patients and you're going to jail. The police already suspect you of killing Lara. This death will seal the deal. Then I'll step in and tell them that I tried to stop you, but you were intent on your mission."

Janessa stunned by the vindictiveness in the woman's tone said, "So, you would kill Elaine just to make the police think that I'm a murderer when you're the one who did it? That doesn't make any sense. What motive would I have to kill a woman I've never met before today? Just like Lara I don't know Elaine. Someone, the police or my friend Margarite will figure it out, so you're bound to be caught sooner or later. "

Terry laughed. It was a harsh cackle filled with evil glee. "Not really. You see after I get rid of her, you'll go to jail. I'll pretend to walk in and catch you killing her. It will be my word against yours and you are a known troublemaker according to Leo and HR. You stick your nose into everything and now everyone will think it's because you were trying to cover your tracks in these deaths."

"But what reason would I have to kill anyone? No one is going to believe it." While Terry was rambling like a mad woman, Janessa watched Elaine. The poor helpless woman bent over the basin and vomited with such force that when she lay back on the bed, her face was bright red with broken blood vessels from the violence of her retching. She was eyeing Terry, and Janessa saw the terror in Elaine's eyes through the tears on her face.

"Now," Terry said. "You're done talking. She's going to die, and you'll go to jail for two murders. Then, I can get close to my father. I've already started that process. He likes me and thinks I'm an excellent nurse. I made sure he knew that I was working when Lara died and that you were capable of murder. Eventually, I'll tell him who I am, and we'll develop a loving father-daughter relationship. Finally, after all these years I'll have my father." Terry looked away momentarily, absorbed by a vision of her perfect life.

This woman is crazy as well as delusional. Janessa mentally went over the details of her last self-defense class. She figured that if she got close enough, she could disarm Terry and take her down. Before she could act, however, everything happened at lightning speed. Terry was still looking at Janessa and gloating when Elaine, though visibly weak, lifted the basin full of vomit and threw it into Terry's face. Janessa had no time to think, she just acted. She flew to Terry's side and grabbed her arms.

The syringe lay on the floor where it had flown out of Terry's hand when the vomit hit her face. She scrambled to get it but slipped in the vomit on the floor. Janessa was faster than Terry and scooped up the syringe and tossed it out of the way. Using a technique she learned in self-defense class, she slammed Terry to the floor face down and pinned her arms behind her back. She put her knee in the center of the woman's back so she couldn't escape.

"Get off me, you bitch! Help! She's trying to kill me. Get her off me," Terry was screaming at the top of her lungs. Suddenly, the room filled with people. At first, they looked puzzled by the two women on the floor.

"Call security," Janessa yelled to Darryl Mintz who was closest. Someone call 911. Terry killed Lara Scutterby and just tried to kill Mrs. Tucker."

Terry was still squirming, trying to get free of Janessa. "She's lying. She's the killer. I was trying to stop her."

Janessa looked over at the security guard standing in front of her looking blank. "Don't just stand there. Don't you have something to secure her wrists? I can't hold her in this position for much longer."

At the no-nonsense tone of her voice, he produced a set of zip ties and secured Terry's wrists. He and Janessa turned a vomit-coated Terry onto her back so she could breathe better.

Mrs. Tucker hoarsely whispered, "She tried to kill me." She pointed at Terry. "I don't know what she was going to put in my arm, but my nurse stopped her."

Janessa pointed to the side of the room. A short distance away lay the syringe. It's over there. I don't know what's in it, but my guess is Sodium Chloride, the same drug she used to kill Lara Scutterby. Did someone call the police?"

"They're almost here," the security guard, who held Terry by her arms said as he began marching her out of the patient cubicle. He gave her a puzzled look. "They said you called a few minutes ago."

Chapter Thirty-Eight

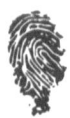

After the police left the emergency department with Terry, a housekeeper went into Elaine's cubicle and cleaned the floor and all the surfaces covered by vomit. The nurses moved Elaine Tucker away from the soiled area and the traumatic memory of her near-death experience. Ashton Hospital provided a counselor for emotional support. Janessa decided not to talk to the counselor after asserting that she was fine, instead opting to continue to care for her patients.

Later, Darryl Mintz examined Elaine. "I have to run some more tests to be sure, Mrs. Tucker, but I suspect you have something called gallstone colic. If I'm not mistaken, you might have a gallstone blocking the duct in your gallbladder. I'll let you know as soon as I have the definitive test results. You have nothing to worry about. We'll take care of the problem and have you back on your feet in no time."

Janessa, standing near her patient heard her comment to Darryl. "After what I just went through with that crazy nurse trying to kill me, a gallstone is nothing." She reached over and patted Janessa's hand. "I can't thank my nurse enough for saving my life. I don't understand why the other nurse wanted to kill me."

Janessa lightly squeezed the woman's hand. "It was your quick thinking that saved the day, Mrs. Tucker. I hate to say it, but I was so glad you chose that moment to vomit."

Everyone laughed, releasing built-up tension, glad everything was over and that it had ended well. Janessa and Mrs. Tucker still had to give their statements to the police, and there would be Terry's trial, but for now, they could relax.

Later that evening, Janessa sat in her kitchen with Margarite and recounted the events of the day. The grapevine in the hospital was rampant, however, as with any event, the facts weren't always accurate. Janessa corrected the misinformation.

"What I want to know is how you managed to call 911. I know Terry didn't stand by while you did that. Someone said that the dispatcher heard everything. They have a recording of the call. The police knew what was happening before they got to the hospital.

Janessa picked up her phone from the table where she'd placed it. Turning the screen toward her friend she said, "My phone is an Android. A feature of that phone is that even if the screen lock is on, you can make an emergency call. See under the box where I put in my password? It says, Emergency Call. Although I couldn't see it, I ran my finger over the screen while pressing it and I connected the call. I started talking louder so that Terry couldn't hear the dispatcher asking me questions about the type of emergency I had. Thankfully, the dispatcher quickly caught on to the fact that I was in trouble. She listened and sent the police. Most calls are automatically recorded so they have all the information that Terry killed Lara and why she did."

"Wow. I'm buying an Android phone. I am so happy she's in jail. Now Pete and I can go on a *real* date and so can you and Lance."

Janessa eyed her friend. "What do you mean a *real* date?"

"I told him I wouldn't date him until you were cleared of Lara's murder. He was fine with that and said he'd wait."

"I'm not sure he believed I'd ever be cleared. When he came here, he was out for my blood."

"Pete said that he had his doubts until you ran into the station when you were being followed. After that day he checked with his uncle and accused him of harassing you, but Leo denied it. At that point, he started to believe that maybe you were telling the truth, and you hadn't killed Lara. With all the other evidence he and Lance collected, they were looking for anyone else who might have done it. Other than you, that is."

Janessa sighed and then took a sip of her tea. "Wonderful. I'm glad he realized I was probably innocent before someone killed me. I've been trying to tell him all along that I never killed anyone. He should have taken me seriously after Brutus and I were thrown into a ditch and my house was trashed."

Margarite patted her hand. "But remember that you didn't report the ditch incident. Anyway, it's over and Lance and I believed in you all along. I heard Lance berate Pete. He told him to open his mind and change his attitude toward you."

"He did?" Janessa asked, sitting back in her chair with a smile on her face. "He criticized him? I wish I could have seen the look on Cranston's face."

"Yes. He told him to change tactics and look elsewhere for the killer. He said there was no way you would hurt anyone, especially a defenseless patient."

At that moment, there was a knock on the door. The women looked at each other. Janessa wasn't expecting anyone. She walked to the front door. After lifting a corner of the curtain on the living room window and looking through, she opened the door. "Mr. Scutterby. I wasn't expecting to see you."

The older gentleman gave her a shaky smile. "I know. I was afraid that if I called you would refuse to see me."

"Come in, please. You know my friend, Margarite?" She gestured to her as they walked into the living area. She saw him nod. She motioned to the sofa and invited Leo Scutterby to take a seat. "What can I do for you?"

He clasped and unclasped his hands without looking down at them and not at Janessa. When he looked up and spoke, she thought she detected a hint that he was holding back tears. He cleared his throat and said, "I want to thank you. I realize now that you tried to save my daughter, Lara. I am so sorry that I accused you of her death. I know my nephew took me at my word when I said you were responsible. He vowed to put you in jail for the rest of your life."

Janessa was speechless. She hadn't been expecting an apology, but it eased the anxiety she'd felt since Lara died. "I.."

"No, let me finish," Leo said, reaching out to take her hands in his gnarled ones. "I am so sorry that Terry, my other daughter found it necessary to hurt people to get to me. I had no idea I had another child. She now knows that I didn't abandon her. I just didn't know she existed. Lara and I had grown apart, but I loved my child. I'll love this daughter too. She took away my Lara, but Terry is still my daughter, and I'll do everything I can to help her."

Janessa looked into his eyes. There was a sheen of tears and sadness. "I'm sorry for your loss. Mr. Scutterby. I wish..."

"I know," he interrupted her. "I know. He stood and surprised Janessa by hugging her then turned to Margarite and did the same. "I'd better go now. The police are going to let me see Terry when the lawyer I hired gets here. Again, thank you for everything."

When he was gone, Janessa and Margarite eyed each other. Margarite handed Janessa her cup of tepid tea. "To happy endings," Janessa said as they clinked their cups together.

Margarite laughed, "Until next time."

About the Author

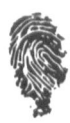

Nanci Race was born in a small city in Western, Massachusetts, the second of six children born to a middle-class family of Native American descent. Her family moved when she was young, to the area known as The Berkshires, also in Western, Massachusetts. She began writing at a young age and even won contests for her poetry when she was in middle school. Although she was encouraged to write by her English teacher, she pursued a career in nursing. Fast forward many years when taking a hiatus from nursing Nanci became the editor of a magazine on the arts. That led to a BA degree in Creative Writing and Literature which she started at Southern Vermont College. After being dually enrolled in Berkshire Community College and Charter Oak State College, two and a half years after starting her journey, she graduated from Charter Oak State in Connecticut.

Nanci returned to nursing for several years, but she was also working on her writing. Eventually many years after completing her BA, she returned to school and within two years had completed her Master of Fine Arts Degree with a concentration in Writing at Lindenwood University in St. Charles Missouri. These days, Nanci is retired from over forty years of nursing and loves spending time with her family, particularly attending her grandchildren's sporting events with her husband. She also is an avid sewist, having spent several years as co-owner of a sewing/tailoring store. In addition to sewing and reading, she enjoys almost all needle arts and travels whenever possible. Nanci currently has stories on the Kindle Vella platform.

Nanci is currently the President of Outreach International Writers, inc. and is a member of Romance Writers of America having served as president of RWA's mystery and suspense chapter, KOD. She is a member of member of Contemporary Romance Writers and a past President of Capital Region RWA.

You can contact Nanci here:

nphill5337817@gmail.com